CLINICAL CARDIOLOGY
Made Easy®

D1571800

CLINICAL CARDIOLOGY
Made Easy®

Ramesh R Rau MD FIAMS CCP
Consultant Physician and Perfusionist
SAL Hospital
Ahmedabad, Gujarat, India

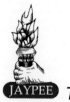

JAYPEE *The Health Sciences Publisher*

New Delhi | London | Philadelphia | Panama

Jaypee Brothers Medical Publishers (P) Ltd

Headquarters

Jaypee Brothers Medical Publishers (P) Ltd
4838/24, Ansari Road, Daryaganj
New Delhi 110 002, India
Phone: +91-11-43574357
Fax: +91-11-43574314
Email: jaypee@jaypeebrothers.com

Overseas Offices

J.P. Medical Ltd
83, Victoria Street, London
SW1H 0HW (UK)
Phone: +44-2031708910
Fax: +44(0)20 3008 6180
Email: info@jpmedpub.com

Jaypee Medical Inc
The Bourse
111 South Independence Mall East
Suite 835, Philadelphia, PA 19106, USA
Phone: +1 267-519-9789
Email: jpmed.us@gmail.com

Jaypee Brothers Medical Publishers (P) Ltd
Bhotahity, Kathmandu
Nepal
Phone: +977-9741283608
Email: kathmandu@jaypeebrothers.com

Jaypee-Highlights Medical Publishers Inc.
City of Knowledge, Bld. 237, Clayton
Panama City, Panama
Phone: +1 507-301-0496
Fax: +1 507-301-0499
Email: cservice@jphmedical.com

Jaypee Brothers Medical Publishers (P) Ltd
17/1-B Babar Road, Block-B, Shaymali
Mohammadpur, Dhaka-1207
Bangladesh
Mobile: +08801912003485
Email: jaypeedhaka@gmail.com

Website: www.jaypeebrothers.com
Website: www.jaypeedigital.com

Inquiries for bulk sales may be solicited at: jaypee@jaypeebrothers.com

Clinical Cardiology Made Easy®

First Edition: **2015**

ISBN 978-93-5152-662-9

Printed at : Samrat Offset Pvt. Ltd.

Dedicated to
All medical students

Preface

There are many good books on cardiology written by well-known cardiologists. The section on cardiology in general medicine textbooks are very concise and often limited. For a medical student, who wishes to understand the basics of heart diseases; and for the practitioner, who would like to brush up on the subject, both of the above options are deterring. Hence, this book aims to fill this vacuum. It is not as long as a treatise on cardiology, but at the same time, it covers all the important aspects adequately.

Another difference is that it is written by a general physician, and so, the emphasis is on the patient and not the investigations; and the approach is always clinical and treatment oriented and not investigation oriented. I have tried to quote Indian figures wherever available, as most Western textbooks do not include them. I have also followed the dictum that common things come first and deserve more mention than rare conditions which may merit just a passing reference. It is also flavored by my personal experience over the years. I have also tried to use an easy language so that it should be a pleasure to read for everybody.

Ramesh R Rau

Acknowledgments

I acknowledge the great role played by my patients in transmitting me the knowledge of cardiology. I thank my wife and daughters for bearing pain who missed me for a long time during writing this book.

Contents

Ischemic Heart Disease

Any book on cardiology should aptly start with this topic as this is the disease which has attracted billions of dollars in research and consequently yielded lot of treatment options and prolonged life in many instances. It is also the most prevalent cardiac disorder encountered in practice.

Ischemic heart disease (IHD) can be classified into angina pectoris, at one end of the spectrum to acute myocardial infarction at the other end. In between is the acute coronary syndrome (ACS).

Angina Pectoris

Epidemiology

The prevalence of IHD is increasing worldwide but we Indians are especially prone to it because of our genetic make-up. It is a disease of affluence as it is seen more in developed world as compared to Third World Countries. In India also the disease is seen more in urban populations than in the rural.

Pathophysiology

IHD can be broadly classified as angina pectoris, unstable angina (ACS) and myocardial infarction (MI). IHD is caused basically by the imbalance between the demand and supply of oxygen-ated blood to the myocardium. When there is 70 percent or more obstruction to blood flow due to atherosclerotic plaques in coronary arteries the blood supply becomes inadequate when the demand is more due to exertion and results in ischemia of the myocardium. This causes effort angina. If there is lesser block but there is thrombosis on it, the supply is not enough to meet basal demands and causes unstable angina. If there is rupture of the plaque of any severity, it then blocks almost the whole lumen and causes total ischemia and results in myocardial infarction. So it can be seen that the atherosclerotic plaque is the villain of the piece. It is caused by the risk factors mentioned below (Fig. 1.1).

As can be seen from the Table 1.1 the first three factors are independent and the others are modifiable.

Classifications

Angina is described according to the severity of exertion required to produce it. The *New York Heart Association classification* is commonly used as follows:

- Class I—No limitation of physical activity (Ordinary physical activity does not cause symptoms).
- Class II—Slight limitation of physical activity (Ordinary physical activity does cause symptoms).
- Class III—Moderate limitation of activity (Patient is comfortable at rest, but less than ordinary activities cause symptoms).
- Class IV—Unable to perform any physical activity without discomfort, therefore severe limitation (Patient may be symptomatic even at rest).

Another system used to describe severity of angina is the Canadian Cardiovascular Society grading scale:

- Class I—Angina only during strenuous or prolonged physical activity.

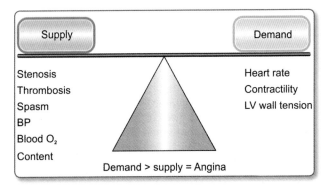

Fig. 1.1: Demand and supply equation of angina

Table 1.1: Risk factors for developing IHD

1. Heredity
2. Male sex
3. Increasing age
4. Diabetes
5. Hypertension
6. Hyperlipidemia
7. Smoking
8. Physical inactivity and obesity
9. High psychological stress
10. a. Homocystine b. High-sensitivity C-reactive protein

- Class II—Slight limitation, with angina only during vigorous physical activity.
- Class III—Symptoms with everyday living activities, i.e. moderate limitation.
- Class IV—Inability to perform any activity without angina or angina at rest, i.e. severe limitation.

Symptoms

Heberden about two and a half centuries ago first described it as follows: There is a disorder of the breast, marked with strong and peculiar symptoms, considerable for the kind of danger belonging to it, and not extremely rare, of which I do not recollect any mention among medical authors. The seat of it, and sense of strangling and anxiety with which it is attended, may make it not improperly be called angina pectoris. The term derives from the Greek *ankhon* 'strangling' and the Latin pectus 'chest'.

Patients of angina usually complain of central chest pain usually located in a diffuse area behind the sternum (Fig. 1.2). It may radiate to left arm, forearm and little finger, to the neck and lower jaw and rarely right arm. The quality of the pain

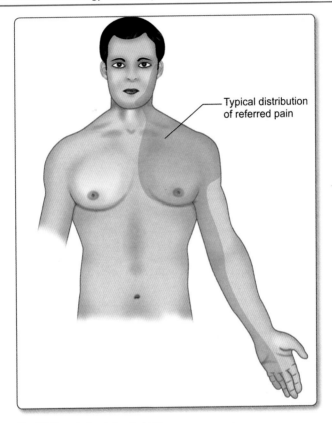

Typical distribution
of referred pain

Fig. 1.2: Sites of referral of anginal pain

is important: It is squeezing type or like a heavy pressure on the chest. The main feature is the association with exertion. It is usually brought on by the same level of activity, e.g. if it comes on after walking 300 meters then it would come on at about the same distance every time. As the disease progresses the level of activity may decrease. Another characteristic feature is that it is immediately relieved by resting. Sometimes the patient complains of pain at say 300 meters. After resting when he starts walking he may walk longer distances without pain. This is described as walking through angina or 'start-up angina'. Sometimes patient may have only dyspnea on exertion. Often pain comes after meals and is called postprandial angina. Often it is brought on by strong emotions like fear, anger, and, etc. or by exposure to intense cold.

What is not angina? Pin-prick pain, pain localized by one finger on the precordium, pain on the outer side of the arm. Pain caused by lifting left arm or stretching left arm.

Signs

There are no specific signs of angina. Patient may be totally normal on examination. There may be associated obesity, hypertension, anxious look, and stains of tobacco on lips, signs of arteriosclerosis like arcus senilis, visible brachial artery pulsations in lower arm, palpable arteries or reduced or absent pulsations of arteries of limbs, bruits over carotids. Also look for anemia or thyrotoxicosis.

Differential Diagnosis

Chest pain of aortic dissection will be accompanied by absent pulses, murmur of AR. Esophageal reflux pain occurs at night, is associated with heavy meals, sour taste in mouth eructation and relieved on sitting up in bed. There may be epigastric burning pain also.

Costochondritis pain occurs on movements of the chest wall and stretching of arms and deep tenderness.

Pneumonia is associated with fever, cough and pleuritic pain.

Investigations

Angina is a clinical diagnosis and the tests are done to confirm or rule out the clinical suspicion. First the ECG should be done ECG is usually normal or may show T wave changes or else it may show old MI pattern. If ECG is taken at the time of chest pain it may show ST depression. More often the patient is seen at some other time and so ECG is often normal. One can reproduce the effort which causes angina by gradually making him exert more and more and watch the ECG and blood pressure. This is done in the treadmill test (TMT). It may show ST depression in multiple leads with or without chest pain. If this occurs at low exercise level it becomes more important or if the changes occur after exercise during the rest period or fails to normalize within 6 minutes. TMT is positive only if the restriction to blow flow is more than 70 percent. Blood pressure may fall in left main disease as a large portion of myocardium is ischemic and transient left ventricular failure occurs. Normal test indicates 'low risk of coronary artery disease (CAD) but not zero risk'.

Echocardiography can also be combined with exercise and it may show wall motion abnormalities. Often it will show change of hypertension in the form of increased wall thickness and diastolic dysfunction.

Stress thallium is another test which will show the perfusion defect during or after the exercise.

Coronary angiography is the gold standard to show the presence and extent of blocks in the epicardial coronary arteries. It will also influence the subsequent treatment modalities (Fig. 1.3).

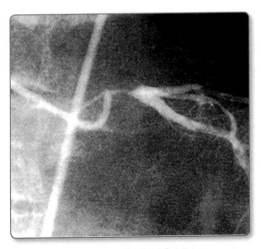

Fig. 1.3: Coronary angiogram showing left main coronary artery stenosis

It is indicated in patients with previous infarction or positive treadmill test or left ventricular (LV) dysfunction seen on echocardiography. It is an invasive procedure with the chance of MI, stroke or other embolism is 1 in 700 (Fig. 1.4).

This is particularly dangerous and life-threatening.

Other investigations should also include the various risk factors which cause angina like blood counts and erythrocyte sedimentation rate (ESR), blood sugars, lipids, electrolytes, uric acid and homocystine. Anemia will aggravate angina. A normal ESR rules out pericarditis. A patient on diuretics may have low K and Mg. Cardiac enzymes are estimated to rule out MI. X-ray chest to look for cardiomegaly due to aneurysm. Widening of mediastinum can be due to dissection.

Treatment

Survival is better with lipid lowering drugs, aspirin and ACE inhibitors. For postinfarction patients, beta-blockers have shown to prolong life in addition.

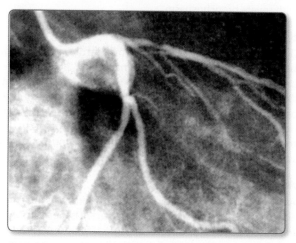

Fig. 1.4: Coronary angiogram showing left anterior descending (LAD) artery proximal block. This can cause massive MI or death (Widow maker artery)

Nitrates

Nitroglycerin causes vasodilation and therefore reduced preload and therefore the wall tension and oxygen requirement of myocardium is reduced so angina is relived. So they will act best when patient is standing or sitting. So angina patient should not lie down but rather sit and take nitroglycerin. It is also a NO donor. Continuous use caused nitrate tolerance or wearing off of its effect. It appears after 24 hours of continuous blood level of the drug. A nitrate-free interval of a few hours restores it efficacy. So isosorbide dinitrates can be taken with eccentric dosing say 8 am, 12 noon and 4 and 8 pm or long- acting isosorbide mononitate can be taken once a day with 16 hours of effect. It can be given to coincide with the angina pattern: A patient with nocturnal angina can be given at night. The most common side effect is headache. This in an indication to stop nitrates.

Calcium Channel Blockers

They reduce afterload by causing arterial dilatation and also reduce myocardial tension and thereby relieve angina. Diltiazem is appropriate alternative to beta-blockers for those with severe bronchospasm.

Beta-blockers

By reducing the heart rate and myocardial wall tension beta-blockers reduce oxygen demand and thereby relieve angina. Bronchospasm may occur with nonselective agents like propranolol. If patient has low heart rate already then agents with intrinsic sympathomimetic action like pindolol or acebutolol may be considered. Claudicaton may occur due to unopposed α adrenergic stimulation causing peripheral vasospasm.

Antiplatelet Drugs

Aspirin prevents platelet aggregation and prevents infarction and death in coronary artery disease. Hence, it is the mainstay of treatment. Clopidogrel can be substituted for those who cannot tolerate aspirin. Though it is marginally better in preventing infarction, its cost is high.

Statins

Statins have been shown to prevent infarction. Bringing down low-density lipoprotein (LDL) cholesterol to less than 70 mg/dL stabilizes atherosclerosis and even regresses it in some persons. Practice guidelines now say that LDL should be brought down below 70 mg/dL irrespective of pretreatment levels.

ACE Inhibitors

ACE inhibitors have also been shown to prevent vascular events in atherosclerotic coronary artery disease. The HOPE trail showed that it also prevents fresh onset diabetes.

Revascularization

All patients with increasing angina, those not controlled on drugs and those with unstable angina should undergo coronary angiogram to evaluate the coronary anatomy and should undergo revascularization if feasible. The latter is done by a balloon which is inflated to press the atherosclerotic plaque against the side of the artery [Percutaneous transluminal coronary angioplasty (PTCA) and subsequently a stent is placed to prevent the artery from abruptly closing (Figs 1.5A and B)].

The second method is to put in place a new conduit to supply blood beyond the blocked segment. This is called coronary artery bypass grafting (CABG). The results of PTCA are evolving and is now comparable to CABG in most cases. The accepted indications for revascularization are left main disease, triple vessel disease and multivessel disease with poor LV function. Restenosis occurs in about 30 percent patients. Stenting lowers the restenosis rate to 20 percent and the newer drug eluting stents reduce the rate to less than 10 percent. These are stents with antiproliferative drugs coated on them which prevents endothelialization and restenosis but with the caveat that dual antiplatelet therapy needs to be taken uninterrupted for possibly lifetime.

CABG increases longevity. Age, cardiac function and the general health are the risk factors. In choosing between PTCA and CABG there is a trade-off: PTCA avoids surgery, a scar, but

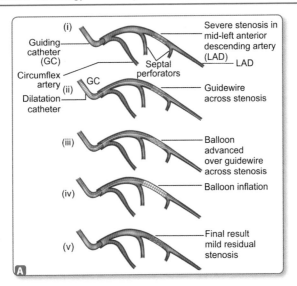

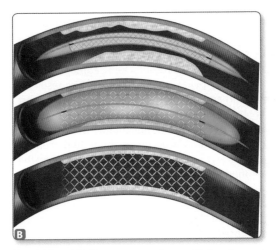

Figs 1.5A and B: Coronary artery disease: (A) Percutaneous transluminal coronary angioplasty (PTCA) and Stenting; (B) Stent deployment after successful PTCA

there is a chance of restenosis requiring another procedure in due course. Diabetics do better with CABG (Fig. 1.6).

Acute Coronary Syndromes

When angina occurs at rest or with minimal activity, often with T changes in ECG without Q waves and sometimes with raised troponin in serum, it is termed acute coronary syndrome (ACS).

Pathophysiology

The atherosclerotic plaques are called vulnerable when it has a thin cover which is prone to rupture and cause platelet aggregation and clot causing further stenosis and reduction in blood flow. These plaques have large, necrotic lipid core with a thin fibrous cap. Inflammatory processes may be involved as evidenced by raised C-reactive protein in ACS. If the thrombus does not occlude fully it caused non ST elevation MI or unstable angina. There can be coronary spasm (Fig. 1.7).

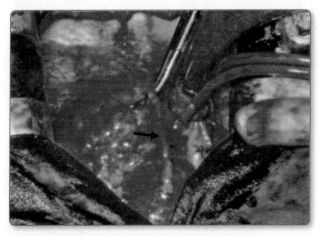

Fig. 1.6: CABG with the graft pointed with arrow

Unstable Angina

Unstable angina is defined as angina pectoris with one of the three features:

1. It occurs at rest or minimal exertion, with prolonged episodes of pain (> 10–15 minutes)
2. It is severe or of new onset (> 2 months)
3. It occurs with a crescendo pattern, is more severe, prolonged or frequent than the previously

   It has a risk of MI or death in 10–40 percent.

NSTEMI

Here there is symptom of unstable angina or minimal symptoms but elevation of troponin or creatine kinase-MB (CK-MB).

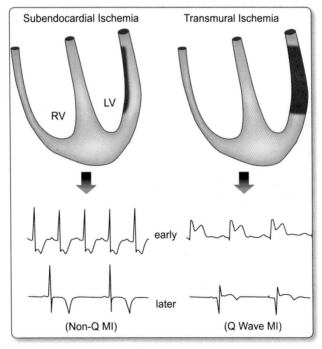

Fig. 1.7: Patterns of myocardial infarction (MI) with arrow

Tight stenosis of a coronary artery with some antegrade flow causes subendocardial ischemia and ST segment depression. If ischemia persists long enough to cause necrosis, there may be T wave inversion the next day. This has been called non-Q MI, or at its outset, non-ST segment elevation MI (NSTEMI). Total occlusion of the coronary artery affects the full thickness of the myocardium, causing ST segment elevation MI (STEMI). With necrosis, Q waves develop (Fig. 1.8).

Presentation
The chest pain is more severe and prolonged than in stable angina pectoris. It is less likely to be relieved by sublingual nitroglycerine. Dyspnea and epigastric discomfort may occur. Nausea, vomiting and sweating may also occur.

Electrocardiogram
The ECG may show ST depression and/or T wave inversion in 30–50 percent of cases.

Biochemical Markers
Troponins are raised in up to 33 percent of cases. CPK-MB may or may not be raised. Hence the troponin is a better essay to employ in ACS setting.

Risk Stratification
Because of the possibility of developing MI, these patients should be classified according to the risk of MI and managed according to the grading of the risk of developing MI. Any patient who has ongoing chest pain, or increasing pain in last 2

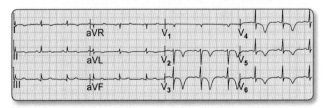

Fig. 1.8: Anterior NSTEMI with symmetric T inversion in anterior leads

days, aged more than 65 years, has more than three risk factors for CAD, has past history of CAD, angina started within 24 hours, has S3 or frank pulmonary edema, ST segment deviation more than 0.5 mm, or has increased cardiac enzymes is at a high-risk and should be admitted and early angiography offered.

Treatment

Goals: (1) control of symptoms, (2) prevention of further episodes of myocardial ischemia.

Medical Therapy

Initially patient is put to strict bed rest with continuous ECG monitoring. Nitrates: Sublingual nitrate tab or spray is given for 3 doses and if not relieved, intravenous nitroglycerine is started at 10 µg/min and increased by 10 µg/min till relieved or the blood pressure falls. Beta-blocker like metoprolol, atenolol or esmolol is given with an aim of bringing heart rate to 50–60 beats per minute. Calcium channel blockers like amlodipine, diltiazem, nifedipine or verapamil are used if nitrates and beta-blockers do not control pain or if beta-blocker is contraindicated.

Antithrombotic treatment: All patients who are not receiving aspirin should be given 325 mg of soluble aspirin dissolved in water. It reduces adverse events by 50–70 percent. Heparin should be added if ACS is diagnosed. Enoxaparin is superior to unfractionated heparin. Addition of clopidogrel reduces cardiac death or MI in 20 percent patients and should be used. Especially if angioplasty or stenting is contemplated clopidogrel should be used about 6 hours prior to it and in the dose of 300–600 mg. After stenting it has been recommended for at least one year and may be indefinitely. However, it also increased the chances of postoperative bleeding by 50 percent in CABG, so if CABG is expected then it is wiser to delay its use till after surgery. If troponins are elevated then glycoprotein IIb/IIa inhibitor should be given before angiography. Abciximab is not effective but tirofiban and eptifibatide are effective. Patients at high risk should be scheduled for angiography and revascularization either by PTCA or CABG.

Acute Myocardial Infarction

Acute myocardial infarction (AMI) is the most dreaded of the cardiac diseases. AMI generally occurs when coronary blood flow decreases abruptly after a thrombotic occlusion of a coronary artery previously narrowed by atherosclerosis. The mortality rate with AMI is approximately 30 percent, with more than half of these deaths occurring before the stricken individual reaches the hospital. Approximately 1 of every 25 patients who survives the initial hospitalization dies in the first year after AMI. Survival is markedly reduced in elderly patients (over age 75); whose mortality rate is 20 percent at 1 month and 30 percent at 1 year after AMI. Myocardial infarction is diagnosed by a triad of chest pain, ECG changes and raised cardiac enzymes.

Pathophysiology

Cigarette smoking, hypertension, and lipid accumulation cause or facilitate vascular injury. When a coronary artery thrombus develops rapidly at a site of vascular injury AMI occurs (Fig. 1.9).

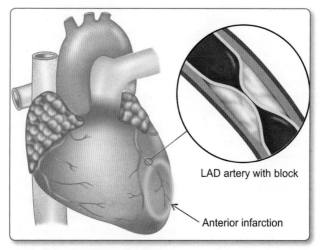

LAD artery with block

Anterior infarction

Fig. 1.9: LAD block resulting in MI

When an atherosclerotic plaque fissures, ruptures, or ulcerates and when conditions (local or systemic) favor thrombogenesis, so that a mural thrombus forms at the site of rupture and leads to coronary artery occlusion. The coronary plaques prone to rupture are those with a rich lipid core and a thin fibrous cap. Thromboxane A_2 is generated at the site causing platelet adhesion and further activation of coagulation cascade. The thrombus so formed occluded the coronary artery. The amount of myocardial damage caused by coronary occlusion depends on (1) the territory supplied by the affected vessel, (2) whether or not the vessel becomes totally occluded, (3) the duration of coronary occlusion, (4) the quantity of blood supplied by collateral vessels to the affected tissue, (5) the demand for oxygen of the myocardium whose blood supply has been suddenly limited, (6) native factors that can produce early spontaneous lysis of the occlusive thrombus, and (7) the adequacy of myocardial perfusion in the infarct zone when flow is restored in the occluded epicardial coronary artery.

Clinical Presentation

In up to 50 percent cases some form of stress like vigorous exercise, Monday morning stress (MI is common on Monday mornings) emotional stress (upsetting life events) or medical or surgical illness precipitates AMI. It commonly occurs early in morning (peak incidence is between 6 am and noon) due to increased sympathetic atone. It is also commoner in winters. The patient has chest pain which is severe often described as the worst pain ever felt in life. It is deep, and is heavy, squeezing or crushing in type. It is similar to the pain of angina pectoris but more severe and prolonged and with a crescendo pattern. It occurs in the central portion of the chest and/or the epigastrium, and on occasion it radiates to the arms. Less common sites of radiation include the abdomen, back, lower jaw, and neck. The frequent location of the pain beneath the xiphoid makes patients' have the common mistaken impression of indigestion, gas or acidity. It is often accompanied by weakness, sweating, nausea, vomiting, anxiety, and a sense of impending doom. The pain may commence when the patient is at rest. When the pain begins during a period of exertion, it does not usually subside with cessation of activity, in contrast to angina pectoris.

Pain may be absent in diabetics, in the elderly, when the presentation is dyspnea. Less common presentations with or without pain, include sudden loss of consciousness, a confusional state, a sensation of profound weakness, the appearance of an arrhythmia, evidence of peripheral embolism, or merely an unexplained drop in arterial pressure.

Signs

The most common finding is an S4 gallop. A soft systolic murmur may be due papillary muscle dysfunction. A soft pericardial rub is heard in first three days in transmural infarction. A loud rub on the other hand is due to pericarditis. Basal rales are important prognostically as described by Killip (Table 1.2). Sinus tachycardia may be present and if it occurs in absence of pain or discomfort, indicates poor LV function. If MI is massive the patient may go in shock with hypotension, perspiration, cold extremities and finally mental obtundation.

ECG

The ST segment of ECG will be depressed in subendocardial ischemia and is the first change in non-ST elevation MI (NSTEMI). This is followed by symmetrical T wave inversion.

Transmural MI (STEMI) will cause ST elevation. In absence of reperfusion ST segment remains elevated for a day and T

Table 1.2: Killip's Class and mortality risk in AMI

Killip Class	Criterion	Mortality risk
I	No rales	6%
II	Rales	17%
III	Pulmonary edema	38%
IV	Cardiogenic shock	81%

inversion occurs. By the time ST segment elevation resolves, Q wave have developed. Infarction may be in anterior, inferior or sometimes posterior walls of the heart (Figs 1.10 to 1.13).

Anterior infarction: This causes ST elevation in chest leads V_1–V_6 and I and aVl and is caused by occlusion of left anterior descending artery (LAD). This is a major vessel supplying most of IVS and LV. And occlusion in its proximal part causes ischemia of IVS and LV, often resulting in LVF. If changes are restricted to V_1 – V_3 it is also called septal infarction.

Inferior infarction: ST elevation in leads II, III, aVf indicates inferior MI. This is caused by occlusion of posterior descending artery PDA branch of right coronary artery in 85 percent and circumflex artery from LCA in the remainder. There can be reciprocal ST depression in anterior (V_1 – V_4) or lateral (I aVl. V_5 – V_6) leads.

Lateral MI: Posterolateral wall is electrophysiologically silent. ST depression in leads V_4–V_6 is usually due to occlusion of LCX artery and a nontransmural infarction results.

True posterior MI: Tall R waves in V_1 – V_2 with ST depression in V_1 – V_3. R waves are also seen in right-sided chest leads: rV1-3. Right ventricular hypertrophy, WPW-A type, and RBBB should be ruled out.

RV infarct: There is ST elevation in right-sided chest leads.

Infarct size: Size of infarcted myocardial mass: In anterior MI the number of leads with ST segment elevation is proportional to the infarct size.

In inferior infarct the sum of ST segment elevations in inferior leads is proportional to infarct size. Reciprocal changes in anterior or lateral leads mean a larger inferior MI.

Bundle branch block—MI can present with new BBB either left or right. With old RBBB ST elevation occurs in V_1 – V_3 leads and indicates proximal LAD occlusion. LBBB obscures MI pattern. Rarely ischemia is indicated by ST elevation in V_4 – V_5 or depression in inferior leads (Figs 1.14 to 1.16).

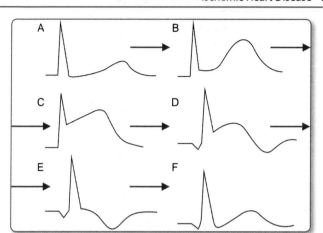

Fig. 1.10: Evolution of acute MI: (A) Normal ECG; (B) Hyperacute T wave change; (C) Marked ST; (D) Q wave, T inverting; (E) Q, T inversion; (F) Q, T upright

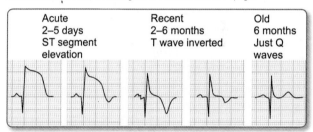

Fig. 1.11: Evolution of ST segments following myocardial infarction

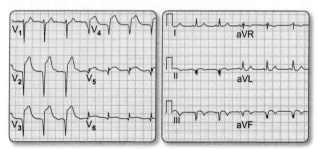

Fig. 1.12: Anterior MI: Presence of Q wave and ST elevation in V_2–V_6

Fig. 1.13: Inferior MI: Q wave, ST elevation, T inversion in II, III and aVf

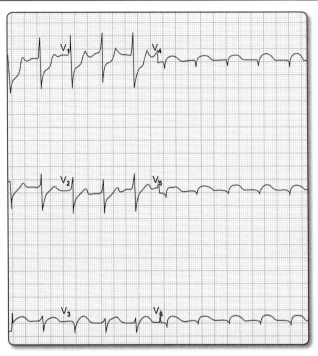

Fig. 1.14: RV infarction: ST elevation in right side V leads: Best in rV_4

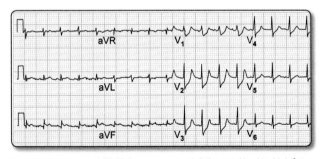

Fig. 1.15: Posterior MI: Tall T, ST depression in V_1–V_3, R/S ratio in V_1 or $V_2 > V_1$. Inferior MI also see inferioposterior

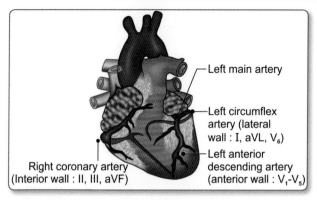

Left main artery

Left circumflex artery (lateral wall : I, aVL, V₆)

Left anterior descending artery (anterior wall : V₁-V₅)

Right coronary artery (Interior wall : II, III, aVF)

Fig. 1.16: Coronary artery anatomy and ECG changes in various leads

Differential Diagnosis

pericarditis has ST elevation but is diffuse and not restricted to inferior or anterior regions, ST segment returns to baseline before T inversion whereas T inversion occurs in MI even when ST is elevated. ST elevation may also occur in LBBB, hyperkalemia, LV, Burgada syndrome. Delta wave of WPW syndrome may appear as Q wave in inferior leads but a short PR clinches the diagnosis. Pseudo Q wave may appear in hypertrophic cardiomyopathy or infiltrative cardiomyopathy.

Cardiac Enzymes

Necrosis of myocardium in an infarction causes the enzymes within to leak out in blood raising their blood levels. Troponin rises as early as 3 hours and lasts for upto 2 weeks. CPK-MB rises by fourth hour and becomes normal by 72 hours. Myoglobin rises by first hour but is nonspecific. The enzymes are tested on admission, at 6, 12 and 24 hours if requires to document a rise (Table 1.3).

Treatment

As soon as a diagnosis of MI is made, the patient should be reassured and kept in bed. He should be transferred to ICU. If there is a delay in shifting thrombolysis may have to be started at home or in casualty department. Nitroglycerin spray or tab is

Table 1.3: Cardiac enzymes in myocardial infarction

	Time of Appearance (hour)		Comment
	Earliest	Peak	
Troponins	3	24	More sensitive than CK-MB Elevation may persist for 7-14 d
CK-MB	4	24	The area under the CK curve is proportional to infarct size. CK-MB/CK >2.5% indicates cardiac injury.
Myoglobin	1–4	6–7	Not specific for heart muscle.

CK, creatine phosphokinase; CK-MB, the myocardium specific band of CK.
'Earlier LDH and its isoforms and SGOT were included. These muscle enzymes are of little use given the better sensitivity and specificity of CK and troponin.

given or IV infusion started if there is no hypotension. For pain relief morphine or tramadol is given with antiemetic phenergan. A tablet of soluble aspirin is given. Clopidogrel in a loading dose of 600 mg is given. A secure IV line is established and blood drawn for investigations. Oxygen is started at 2–4 L/min and continued for 1 day or 2 days. Those going for angioplasty may be given IIb/IIa inhibitor as well. Statins are given as 40–80 mg atorvastatin.

A. *NSTEMI:* Here the results are poor with thrombolysis and so they are treated with antithrombotics (aspirin, clopidogrel, IIB/IIIa inhibitor and heparin) and when stable and free from pain, taken for angiography and angioplasty usually the next day.

B. *STEMI:* If the patient comes within 3 hours of chest pain he should be taken up for primary angioplasty. If he presents later he is thrombolysed. If shifting a patient to a cardiology set-up is going to take more than 60 minutes, it is better to thrombloyse.

Thrombolysis: This is indicated in STEMI or MI with new LBBB or an inability to reach cath lab in a tertiary care center for angiography within 2 hours. It is contraindicated in persons more than 75 years of age, active peptic ulcer, recent surgery, recent

CPR with chest contusion, recent stroke, bleeding diathesis or on warfarin, severe uncontrolled hypertension, recent intracranial or spinal surgery or trauma. The complications are bleeding from puncture site and hemorrhagic stroke, systemic emboli, allergic reaction (Fig. 1.17).

Mechanism: Clot formation is accompanied by fibrinolytic system activation as clot cannot be allowed to propagate and must be removed eventually. Plasminogen in plasma is converted to plasmin by Plasminogen activators .These include naturally occurring substances, t-PA, urokinase and streptokinase. Plasmin breaks down fibrin strands in the clot to fibrinogen degradation products. It also digests circulating fibrinogen and thereby produces a hypocoagulable state. SK is nonspecific in that it degrades both fibrinogen in circulation and in the clot. Others are fibrin specific so that only fibrinogen in clot is lysed. t-PA is better than SK.

Reperfusion: About 55–65 percent have reperfusion following thrombolysis. It is marked by a reduction in chest pain and normalizing of ST segments in ECG. Occasionally reperfusion

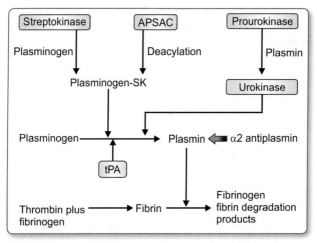

Fig. 1.17: Mechanism of coronary thrombolysis

Table 1.4: Risk of death from myocardial infarction and patient selection for reperfusion therapy

Highest risk, immediate reperfusion therapy is indicated	Anterior MI Large inferior MI Inferior MI and possible RV infarction MI with new bundle branch block
Lower risk, consider emergency reperfusion based on other clinical features	NSTEMI with persistent pain Small inferior MI in a patient who is not a good candidate for reperfusion
Clinical features that increase the risk of MI, and would favor reperfusion therapy	Heart failure (Killip class II-IV) Prior MI History of heart failure RV infarction syndrome diabetes

Abbreviations: MI—Myocardial infarction; RV—Right ventricular.

arrhythmias occur—the commonest is a short run of accelerated idioventricular rhythm which does not require any treatment. VT or VF is rare. Twenty-five percent will occlude if the stenosis is not relieved (Table 1.4).

Subsequent Management

A. *Antithrombotic therapy:* Aspirin and heparin are started with thrombolysis. Heparin can be delayed if SK is used ad here is a hypocoagulable state produce already. Heparin is monitored with APTT which should be kept 11/2–2 times control.

B. *Beta-blockade:* IV atenolol or metoprolol is used, followed by tablets. It reduces infarct size, prevents sudden cardiac death, reinfarction. It is contraindicated in presence of S_3 gallop, shock, pulmonary edema, heart block, asthma , peripheral ischemia, PR > 24 sec, and heart rate < 60 beats per minute.

The use of beta-blockers in the acute phase of MI is summarized in Table 1.5. If bronchospasm is a concern, use the short-acting agent, esmolol, 5–25 µg/kg minute (Table 1.5).

C. Heparin is given immediately after tPA or later after SK. It should be especially given with large infarct, those slow to mobilize or with heart failure. Low molecular weight heparins are preferred as they have shown better results with lesser side effects like bleeding.

Table 1.5 : Beta-blocker therapy for acute MI

Patient selection	Acute MI, <12 h from the onset of pain
Contraindications	1. Heart failure (diffuse rales) 2. Heart rate < 60 beats per minute 3. Heart block (PR interval > 24 sec) 4. Systolic blood pressure < 90 mmHg 5. Asthma or obstructive lung disease with wheezing
Metoprolol	5 mg IV at 5 min intervals for heart rate of 60 beats per minute and BP of 100 mmHg
	100 mg PO qid for 48 hr Then 100 mg PO bid
Atenolo	5 mg IV over 5 min, repeat in 10 minutes (no second dose if heart rate or blood pressure decrease
	Then 50 mg PO 10 minutes later Then 50 mg PO bid
Benefits	Blunts catecholamine effect, lowering MVO_2 and thus, infarct size. ST segment elevation may resolve
	Survival may also be improved by prevention of ventricular fibrillation or LV rupture

Abbreviations: bid—Twice daily; LV—Left ventricular; MI—Myocardial infarction; MVO_2—Maximal venous oxygen consumption; PO—Orally; qid—Four times daily

D. IV nitrates are used for continued chest pain, and LVF. It improves LV function, reduces infarct size. Hypotension if occurs can be corrected by supine position, elevation of legs.

E. *ACE inhibitor:*This is shown to limit infarct size, improve survival and LV function. Best results are seen when started within 24 hours. Captopril is started at 6.25 mg and dose gradually built up to 25 mg tds. Enalapril and ramipril and perindropril are also useful. Hypotension may occur.

F. Calcium channel blockers have not been shown to be useful and should not be used. Diltiazem has been shown to be useful in one trial.

Table 1.6: Angiotensin-converting enzyme inhibition after myocardial infarction

Patient selection	1. Anterior MI 2. MI complicated by heart failure 3. LVEF <30%
Contraindication	Systolic pressure < 100 mmHg known renal artery stenosis, prior reaction to ACE inhibition
Drugs and oral dose (begin on day 1 of MI)	Captopril 12.5–50 mg bid Enalapril 5–20 mg bid Lisinopril 2.5–10 mg bid Ramipril 2.5–5 mg bid Perindropril 2 mg

Postinfarct Management

Those who are thrombolysed should be subjected to submaximal treadmill test to document any ischemia. If positive they should be taken for angiography and then revascularization (Table 1.6).

A. *Diet:* Patients have to be explained the importance of fat restricted diet and weight loss. They should quit smoking.

B. Alcohol is permitted in moderation bearing in mind the weight loss regime.

C. *Work and exercise:* Patients can return to work about 4 to 6 weeks after the MI. If possible work tensions should be reduced or a work with lesser burden chosen. Exercise like regular walking for 30 minutes a day must be encouraged. A treadmill test showing not ECG changes at a heart rate of about 120 beats per minute is good for doing most routine activities safely.

Secondary Prevention

A. Aspirin should be taken 75–150 mg per day probably indefinitely. It has been shown to reduce mortality and reinfarction.

B. Beta-blockers: Also reduce major adverse cardiovascular events.

C. *ACE inhibitor:* Ramipril should be given in the largest tolerated dose 5 mg bd as HOPE trial has shown reduction in mortality and reinfarction.

D. Statins should be continued too to keep LDL below 70 mg/dL, triglycerides below 150 and HDL above 40 mg/dL.

Complication of MI

Left ventricular failure can occur if a large part (40%) of myocardium has infarcted. RV failure occurs if RV infarct is large. If there is persistent hypotension <80 mmHg, pulmonary edema and cold clammy extremities and low urine output and altered sensorium, the condition is called cardiogenic shock. Cardiogenic shock occurs in about 5–7 percent when 80 percent of myocardium is infarcted and the mortality is about 40 percent. Shock generally occurs within 3 days of MI. The treatment of this is reperfusion. The patient must be taken for angioplasty with best results occur if done within 4 hours of MI. Intra-aortic balloon pump (IABP) will help buy time for reperfusion.

LV aneurysm can develop if there is infarct thinning.

LV clot can develop on the infarct surface as it is hypokinetic or akinetic (Fig. 1.18). This can embolize to any organ of the body.

VSD occurs if the interventricular septum undergoes necrosis. It develops in first week of MI. Biventricular failure follows. Mortality is high (50–85%) unless treated surgically.

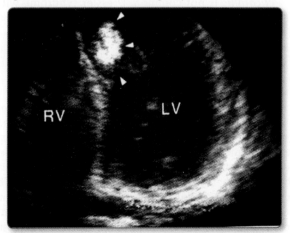

Fig. 1.18: Echocardiogram showing a clot in LV after anterior MI

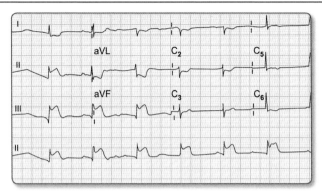

Fig. 1.19: AV block in inferior MI

Mitral regurgitation occurs due to LV dilation or chordal or papillary muscle rupture. Papillary rupture occurs in 1 percent and mostly with inferior MI. There is a loud systolic murmur and pulmonary edema. Echocardiography is diagnostic.

Heart block is temporary in inferior infarct but often permanent in anterior MI. In the later situation a pacemaker may be required (Fig. 1.19).

Pericarditis is not common. Dressler syndrome with pericarditis, pleural effusion, fever, high ESR is not uncommon, it responds well to NASIDs. Many of the above complications need surgical correction.

Intracardiac thrombus often develops in large anterior infarcts. A part of the clot can embolize and cause systemic embolism in brain or limbs.

Cardiac rupture can cause tamponade also rarely. *Arrhythmias:* Malignant ventricular arrhythmias and sudden cardiac death is also known. A serum potassium level is inversely proportional to development of ventricular ectopics and VT. For decades ventricular ectopics were treated vigorously but the CAST trial showed that there were more sudden cardiac deaths in spite of suppression of VPCs. Thus, beta-blockade is better as it prevents SCD even if VCs are not suppressed. For VT beta-blocker or if not controlled amiodarone can be used. The MADIT trial suggests use of automatic implantable cardioverter-defibrillator (AICD) to prevent SCD.

Hypertension: The Silent Killer

Hypertension is the second most prevalent disease and hence deserves to be given due weightage. It is a modifiable risk factor for cardiovascular disease, and if left untreated, causes devastating effects like stroke, myocardial infarction, renal and peripheral vascular disease.

Epidemiology

Cardiovascular diseases caused 2.3 million deaths in India in the year 1990; this is projected to double by the year 2020. Hypertension is directly responsible for 57 percent of all stroke deaths and 24 percent of all coronary heart disease deaths in India. It is also a disease of affluence. Hypertension is present in 25 percent urban and 10 percent rural subjects in India. The estimated total number of people with hypertension in India in 2000 was 60.4 million males and 57.8 million females and is projected to increase to 107.3 million and 106.2 million respectively in 2025.

About 50 million Americans are hypertensive. According to Framingham study for normotensive persons at 55 years of age there is a 90% probability of developing hypertension at some time during life.

Apart from the huge numbers one has to remember that we are treating hypertension not to bring down the numbers but to prevent endorgan damage especially to heart, brain and kidneys. This should be emphasized to the patients too, to make them realize the importance of treating hypertension to goals.

Definition

So when do we treat high blood pressure? Hypertension in adults age 18 years and older is defined as systolic blood pressure (SBP) of 140 mmHg or greater and/or diastolic blood pressure (DBP) of 90 mmHg or greater. This should be based on the average of two or more blood pressure readings taken in sitting position and at least on two visits after an initial screening. The classification of blood pressure is shown in Table 2.1. Apart from the pressure presence of target organ damage should be noted. The risk of CVD doubles for every 20/10 mmHg above 115/75 mmHg. Treating hypertension lowers risk of stroke by 40 percent, ischemic heart disease by 25 percent and heart failure by 50 percent. The rule of halves: Half of hypertensives are undetected, half of those detected are untreated, half of those treated are inadequately controlled. Those in prehypertension stage have double the chance of developing hypertension.

Etiology

About 90–95 percent of hypertension is primary with no cause found. In the remaining, it is called secondary hypertension denoting the presence of some other disease leading to hypertension. The causes of secondary hypertension are given in Tables 2.2 and 2.3 and shown in Figure 2.1. Every patient should be evaluated clinically and if secondary cause is suspected, relevant investigations must be done.

Table 2.1: Classification of hypertension

Category	Systolic (mmHg)		Diastolic (mmHg)
Optimal	<120	and	<80
Normal	<130	and	<85
High-normal/ Prehypertension	130–139	or	85–89
Hypertension Stage 1 Stage 2 Stage 3	140–159 160–179 >180	or or or	90–99 100–109 >110
Isolated systolic hypertension Grade 1 Grade 2	140–159 >160	and and	<90 <90

Table 2.2: Keith and Wagner's grading of hypertensive retinopathy

Grade 1	Thickening and tortuosity of arteries showing 'silver wiring' appearance
Grade 2	Grade 1 changes plus arteriovenous nipping
Grade 3	Grade 2 changes plus flame-shaped (superficial) hemorrhages and cotton wool exudates
Grade 4	Grade 3 changes plus papilledema

Stress can increase blood pressure but that is usually a rise in systolic pressure, it is short-lived and comes to normal once the stress is over or if the person rests.

Sex

Systolic BP increases with age. This increase is more marked in men than in women until women reach menopause, when their BP rises more sharply and reaches levels higher than in men. The prevalence of hypertension is higher in men than in women younger than 55 years but is higher in women older than 55 years. The prevalence of hypertensive heart disease probably follows the same pattern.

Age

BP increases with age, as does the prevalence of hypertensive heart disease, which is affected by the severity of BP increase.

Symptoms

It should be stressed again and again that hypertension per se causes no symptoms. Very often patient is unaware of it. Hence, hypertension is called the silent killer. If the pressure is very high like >200/120 mmHg then headache has been observed. This headache is usually in the occipital region, dull, constant. The patient may have symptoms due to complications like palpitations, dyspnea, etc. Epistaxis may be associated with severe hypertension. Patients may have palpitations in case of arrhythmias or dyspnea in case LV failure sets in. Patients may complain of chest pain due to associated coronary heart disease.

Signs

There are no sign specific to hypertension. There may be associated signs of atherosclerosis. There may be signs of left ventricular hyper-trophy. Of patients with hypertension, 15–20 percent develops LVH. The risk of LVH is increased 2-fold by associated obesity. Thyromegaly arterial narrowing on retinoscopy, bruits over renal arteries, aorta or carotids, or femroals, S_4 sound loud S_2 (A_2), lower BP in lower limbs than upper limbs and delayed or absent femoral pulses in coarctation of aorta. Arcus senilis, xanthalasma and xanthomas suggest elevated blood lipids. Bruits may be heard over stenosed arteries in neck, limbs or abdomen. The retina will show thickening of arteries and hemorrhages and exudates (dots and blots) see adjoining Figure 2.1.

Funduscopic examination is important to detect retinopathy.

Measurement of Blood Pressure

The patient should be relaxed when measuring blood pressure. He should be seated for at least 30 minutes and should not have had a coffee or tea or smoked in last 30 minutes. Blood pressure should be measured in sitting position and a raised pressure should be rechecked in other arm. An elevated reading should also be confirmed at two other visits.

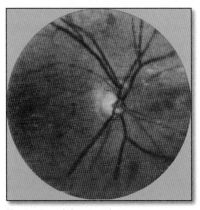

Fig. 2.1: Retinal changes in hypertension

Laboratory Evaluation of Hypertension

Laboratory tests are done to (i) check any target organ damage due to hypertension, (ii) assess risk of CVD which might define the prognosis and guide treatment. (iii) to detect cause of hypertension if any. Hence complete blood counts should be done. Renal failure will result in anemia. Urine exam will show albuminuria, deposits and casts in renal failure, sugar in diabetes. Blood urea and creatinine will show the renal status. Serum potassium will be low in hyperaldosteronism when not on diuretics. Low potassium during treatment with diuretics especially thiazides, is also a cause of arrhythmias and sudden cardiac death.

Lipid profile should be done to document baseline levels as a CVD risk factor. Blood glucose will be high in secondary causes of hypertension like Cushing's syndrome, pheochromocytoma and primary aldosteronism.

Serum calcium and phosphorus is a screen for hyper-parathyroidism a potential cause for secondary hypertension. Uric acid may rise with diuretic therapy and in renal failure so a baseline test is useful.

ECG is a must. But, it detects LV hypertrophy in only about 50 percent of cases. The earliest sign of LVH is left an atrial abnormality: A biphasic P in V_1. Due to hypertension there is increased LV end diastolic pressure leading to increase in LA and LA appendage size and thickness. This is reflected in the ECGs. This implies chronicity and correlates with LV diastolic dysfunction. There can be conduction abnormalities like LBBB, ST changes of ischemia.

X-ray chest is a must to detect LV enlargement, and coarctation where there is dilated ascending aorta and rib notching due to enlarged intercostals arteries.

Further testing is done if secondary hypertension is suspected. JNC 7 has recommended that "more extensive testing for identifiable causes is not generally indicated unless BP control is not achieved."

Echocardiography is now a recommended tool to detect and quantify left ventricular hypertrophy (LVH). Proper treatment will cause the hypertrophy to regress. With uncontrolled hypertension, LVH is risk factor for CVD. It may also show evidence of diastolic dysfunction in the form of reversed E:A ratio. If there is failure, systolic dysfunction will be evident in the form of enlarged LV, low ejection fraction and LA dilatation, and mitral insufficiency (Figs 2.2 to 2.5).

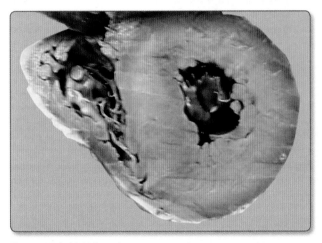

Fig. 2.2: Marked LVH due to hypertension seen in an autopsy specimen

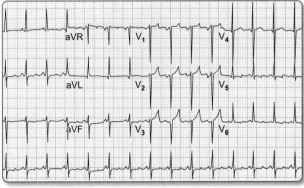

Fig. 2.3: ECG of a 47-year-old man with a long-standing history of uncontrolled hypertension showing left atrial enlargement and left ventricular hypertrophy

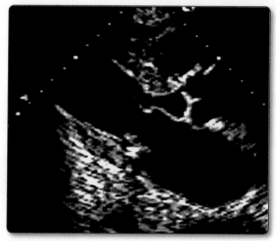

Fig. 2.4: Two-dimensional echocardiogram of a 70-year-old woman (parasternal long axis view) showing concentric left ventricular hypertrophy

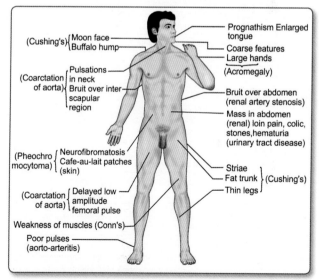

Fig. 2.5: Causes of secondary hypertension

Secondary Hypertension

Causes of secondary hypertension are listed in Table 2.3 and shown in the Figure 2.5.

Table 2.3: Causes of secondary hypertension

Secondary Hypertension	Clinical picture	Lab evaluation
Renal artery stenosis	HBP under age 20 years Abdominal or flank bruit New onset or worsening HT in older patient with increasing creatinine	Renal Doppler, MR angiography, Captopril augmented renal scan Angiography
Chronic renal parenchymal disease	Clinical setting	Creatinine clearance
Pheochromocytoma	Paroxysmal HBP, headache, flushing, tachycardia	Urinary VMA CT scan of abdomen
Coarctation of aorta	Young hypertensive, decreased BP in lower limbs, decreased or delayed femoral pulses	CT scan chest
Hyperaldosteronism	Hypokalemia, possible hypernatremia	CT scan of adrenal glands
Hyperparathyroidism	Kidney stones, weakness, lethargy, osteoporosis	Serum calcium and PTH level
Hyperthyroidism	Systolic HBP, heat intolerance, weight loss, tremors, new AF	TSH level
Hypothyroidism	Diastolic HBP, fatigue, weight gain, weakness	TSH level
Cushing's syndrome	Typical habitus	Dexamethasone suppression test
Sleep apnea	Obesity, thick neck, snoring, daytime somnolence	Sleep study
Drug side effects	Erythropoietin, cyclosporine, NASIDs, COX2 inhibitors, birth control pills, steroids, appetite suppressants, pseudoephedrine, nicotine, MAO inhibitors, amphetamines, testosterone	

Treatment

Table 2.4 showing the risk of patients with hypertension.

That treatment of hypertension is very effective is beyond any doubt. A large meta-analysis has shown that 5–6 mmHg reduction in diastolic pressure will result in 14 percent reduction of coronary heart disease and a whopping 42 percent reduction in cerebrovascular incidents over a 5-year period. That has been followed by another landmark trial showing a massive benefit in reducing systolic hypertension in elderly.

Table 2.4: Risk stratification of patients with hypertension

		Blood pressure (mmHg)		
Stage	Other risk factors and disease history	Stage 1	Stage 2	Stage 3 (severe hypertension)
		SBP 140–159 or DBP 90–99	SBP 160–179 or DBP 100–109	SBP ≥ 180 or ≥ DBP 110
I	No other risk factors	Low risk	Medium risk	High risk
II	1–2 risk factors[a]	Medium risk	Medium risk	Very high risk
III	3 or more risk factors or TOD[b] or diabetes	High risk	High risk	Very high risk
IV	ACC[c]	Very high risk	Very high risk	Very high risk

Risk strata (typical 10 years risk of stroke or myocardial infarction)

Low risk = Less than 15 percent

Medium risk = About 15–20 percent

High risk = About 20–30 percent

Very high risk = 30 percent or more

[a]See Table 2.5

[b]TOD: Target organ damage see Table 2.5

[c]ACC: Associated clinical condition, including clinical cardiovascular disease or renal disease see Table 2.5

Goals

The blood pressure should be lowered to less than 130/85 mmHg in all patients at all ages. For those with diabetes and renal disease the goal is less than 125/75. For very elderly patients more than 80 years, it should be less than 150/80. Effective blood pressure is required to delay or reverse complications and this reduces the overall risk of the person without affecting the quality of life.

The First Step is Lifestyle Modification

This involves dietary modification firstly. A low salt diet reduces blood pressure. Indian diet is loaded with salt to the tune of 10–15 g/day. A diet of 3–6 g salt is recommended , which leads to a reduction of about 2–8 mmHg. Table salt (sodium chloride) is the most obvious source of sodium in your diet. Just one teaspoon of salt contains 2,000 mg of sodium, which is just a little less than the entire amount you should have in one day. The salt you add when cooking or at the table is only part of total sodium intake. Even natural foods such as milk, meat and vegetables contain sodium. A cup of milk contains 375 mg of sodium. A half cup of cottage cheese has 475 mg. A glass of tomato juice has 441 mg. Foods that tend to be higher in sodium are soups, soy sauce, chili sauce, mustard, pickles and relishes, processed cheese and cheese spread, baking powder, baking soda and most baked goods, which contain these ingredients, cured ham, sausages and luncheon meats, salted nuts, chips and other snack foods, any food additive with the word "sodium" (sodium benzoate, a preservative; sodium phosphate, an emulsifier and stabilizer).

A high potassium diet also reduces blood pressure. So a diet rich in fruits and green leafy vegetables rich in potassium, such as bananas, oranges, avocados, and tomatoes should be advocated for patients with normal renal function. Unless you have kidney disease, you should eat about 3,500 mg of potassium each day. A baked potato has 875 mg. A glass of prune juice has 704. A cup of yogurt has 578.

What about salt substitutes? This may be helpful, but keep this in mind:

- Some salt substitutes contain a mixture of salt and other compounds. To get that familiar salty taste, you may end up using more salt substitute and not reducing your sodium intake at all.

- Potassium chloride is a common ingredient in salt substitutes. Too much potassium can be harmful for people with kidney problems. Extra potassium may be hazardous when people with high blood pressure or heart failure take certain medications that may cause the kidneys to retain potassium (Potassium—based salt substitutes have a bitter taste if they are cooked).

Instead of salt or salt substitutes, to enhance the flavor of food by using herbs and spices, flavored vinegars or lemon juice.

Regular aerobic exercise: Walking, running, swimming or cycling regularly for 30 minutes a day for 5 days a week has been shown to reduce BP by 4–9 mmHg. It also improves cardiovascular function favorably. Isometric and strenuous exercise should be avoided.

Weight reduction: Each 10 kg weight loss is associated with 5–20 mmHg pressure reduction.

Avoid drugs like NASIDs, steroids, contraceptive pills which can increase blood pressure.

Drugs

Formerly a 'step-care approach' was advocated wherein first a diuretic was started, then a beta-blocker was added as step two, calcium channel blocker was step three and ACE inhibitors and others as step four.

This step care is no longer advocated and any drug can be started and certain drugs in particular situations are favored. JNC 7 recommends to start 2 drugs one of them being diuretics for a pressure which is 20/10 mmHg above the goal (Table 2.4).

All drug classes are equally effective in lowering blood pressure individually (TOMHS study). Combining drugs from different classes is advantageous as that not only lowers blood pressure more effectively but the side effects of one is counterbalanced by the other. For example, combining beta-blocker, which reduces heart rate, with a calcium channel blocker which increases heart rate is obviously beneficial.

Similarly, the potassium loss due to diuretic is counter balanced by the hyperkalemic propensity of ACE inhibitors. Thus judicious combination of two classes and often three is necessary to effectively bring down the blood pressure.

Diuretics

Thiazides and indapamide: These have actions like dilatation of resistance vessels due to calcium activated potassium channels and a minor effect due to diuresis. Indapamide is calcium antagonist. The side effects to watch are hypokalemia (in less than 1%) and hyponatremia especially in elderly, hypotension, hyperglycemia in some, hyperuricemia (which is innocuous), hypertriglyceridemia and hypercholesterolemia in 2.5 percent of cases, general weakness, lethargy. They should not be used in renal failure (creatinine more than 1.5 mg/dL) and those having gout or hyperuricemia. Indapamide has minimal metabolic side effects (Table 2.5).

In 20 percent of patients they are inadequate or inappropriate. They require drugs from other classes of compounds (Table 2.6).

Beta-blockers

These are most widely-used agents. They are most effective in young patients, those with angina or postmyocardial infarction. However recent trials have not shown mortality benefit with beta-blocker especially atenolol. This was true in trials of atenolol with diuretics. They are also less effective than calcium channel blockers in preventing stroke and new onset diabetes. But it is not appropriate to extrapolate this data on atenolol to other selective beta-blockers. Agents with intrinsic sympathomimetic activity and highly selective beta-blockers such as Nebivolol and bisoprolol have minimal metabolic adverse effects. They are have compelling role in young people, women with childbearing potential, those intolerant to ACE inhibitors or ARBs and those with increased sympathetic drive. They are contraindicated in asthma and COPD (Flow chart 2.1 and Table 2.7).

Table 2.5: Guidelines for selecting the most appropriate antihypertensive drugs

Class of drugs	Definite indications	Possible indications	Definite contraindications	Relative contraindications
Diuretics	– Heart failure – Elerly patients – Systolic hypertension	– Diabetes	– Gout	– Dyslipidemia
Beta blockers	– Angina – Post-myocardial infarction – Tachyarrhythmia Heart failure	– Pregnancy – Diabetes	– Asthma and chronic pulmonary disease – Heart block[a]	– Dyslipidemia – Physically active – Peripheral vascular disease
CCB's	– Angina – Elderly – Systolic hypertension – Diabetes	– Peripheral Vascular disease – CVA	– Heart block[b]	– Congestive heart failure[c]
ACE inhibtor	– Heart failure – Left ventricular dysfunction – Post-myocardial infarction – Significant proteinuria – Diabetes	– CVA	– Pregnancy and lactation – Bilateral renal artery stenosis – Hyperkalemia	– Moderate renal failure (Creatinine > 3 mg/dL)
Angiotensin Receptors Blockers (ARBs)	– ACE inhibitor induced cough	– Heart failure – CVA	– Pregnancy and lactation – Bilateral renal artery stenosis – Hyperkalemia	– Moderate renal failure (Creatinine levels 3 mg/dL)
Alpha blockers	– Prostatic hypertrophy	– Glucose intolerance – Dyslipidemia	–	– Orthostatic hypertension – Congestive heart failure

[a]Grade 2 or 3 atrioventricular block
[b]Grade 2 or 3 atrioventricular block with verapamil or diltiazem
[c]Verapamil or diltiazem

Table 2.6: Diuretics

Diuretic	Trade name	Usual dose range
Hydrochlorothiazide (HCTZ)	Aquazide, Xenia	12.5 mg daily
Chlorthalidone	Hythalton, Hydrazide	12.5–25 mg daily
Indapamide	Natrilix	2.5 mg daily
Potassium sparing		
HCTZ + Triamterene	Ditide	25 + 50 mg daily
HCTZ + Amiloride	Biduret	50 + 5 mg/day
Spironolactone	Aldactone	25–100 mg daily
Torsemide	Dytor, Tide,	5–10 mg daily
Furosemide	Lasix	20–40 mg/day
Amiloride + Furosemide	Amifru	5 + 40 mg/day

Flow chart 2.1: Beta-adrenoceptor blocking drugs

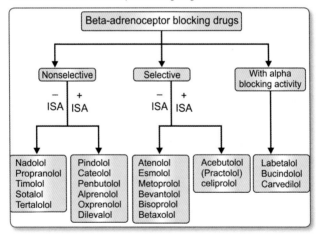

Calcium Channel Blockers

a. Dihydropyridines: Nifedipine, amlodipine
b. Nondihydropyridines: Diltiazem, verapamil

Table 2.7: Beta-blockers

Blockers range	Trade name	Usual dosage
Propranolol*	Inderal®, Ciplar Inderal® LA	20–120 mg BID 60–240 mg daily
Nadolol*	Corgard®, generic	20–160 mg daily
Timolol*	Blocadren®, generic	5–20 mg BID
Atenololº	Tenormin®, Betacard	25–100 mg daily
Metoprololº	Betaloc®, Lopressor®, generic	25–100 mg BID
	Betaloc® SR, Lopressor® SR	100–200 mg daily
Acebutolol^	Sectral®, Monitan®, generic	100–400 mg daily
Oxprenolol^	Trasicor® Slow Trasicor®	20–160 mg BID, 80–320 mg daily
Pindolol*^	Visken®, generic	5–15 mg
Labetalol*ª	Trandate®	100–400 mg BID

* Nonselective || º selective || ^ partial agonist || ª alpha blocker

Besides antihypertensive properties, they also have anti-anginal effects and are devoid of metabolic effects. Verapamil and diltiazem also reduce heart rate and have negative isotropic effects. They are recommended for the elderly hypertensives with isolated systolic hypertension. The findings of the recent ASCOT-BPLA (blood pressure lowering arm) study show that an antihypertensive drug regimen starting with amlodipine (adding perindopril as required) is better than one starting with atenolol (adding thiazide as required) in terms of reducing the incidence of all types of cardiovascular events and all-cause mortality, and risk. Short-acting dihydropyridines like nifedipine should be avoided as they can cause tachycardia, increased oxygen demand and vasodilatation. Amlodipine is better as it is long-acting and has no effects on heart rate and contractility and can be used in heart failure. Edema is a troublesome side effect of this group.

Angiotensin Converting Enzyme Inhibitors (ACE inhibitors)

Enalapril, lisinopril, ramipril, perindopril, Quinapril, are safe and good antihypertensive agents. They reduce mortality and morbidity after MI. In diabetic they reduce and prevent progression of renal disease .The HOPE trial (a primary prevention trial) showed that in high and average risk individuals, use of ramipril reduced overall 61 mortality and cardiovascular endpoints, even with small reductions in blood pressure. They have no metabolic side effects. The commonest side effect is a dry irritating cough without expectoration and which is often at night. They can cause angioedema. These two side effects are due to accumulation of bradykinin. They cause a rise in serum potassium, hence are suitable for use with diuretics except potassium sparing ones. They raise creatinine in patient with bilateral renal artery stenosis and hence are contraindicated.

Angiotensin Receptor Blockers

These are losartan, candesartan, valsartan, irbesartan and telmisartan and olmisartan. In the LIFE trial, losartan was better than atenolol in reducing the frequency of the primary composite endpoint of stroke, myocardial infarction and cardiovascular death marginally. They may increase the rates of myocardial infarction despite their beneficial effects on reducing blood pressure. However, this needs further evaluation. These drugs have many features in common with ACE inhibitors, but do not cause an accumulation of bradykinin. Consequently, cough and angioedema are much less likely to occur than with ACE inhibitors.

Alpha-blockers

Alpha-blockers such as prazosin, terazosin and doxazosin—effectively reduce blood pressure both as monotherapy and in combination. They improve insulin sensitivity and have no adverse effects on lipids. They are best suited for elderly, males with benign prostatic hyperplasia. The main side effect is postural hypotension. Hence, the dose should be gradually titrated upwards. They are also useful in chronic renal failure, peripheral vascular diseases, and metabolic disorders. If heart failure develops they should be withdrawn.

Other Drugs

Centrally acting drugs have been in use for several years. In particular, methyldopa remains an important agent for the treatment of hypertension in pregnancy. Clonidine, though a potent antihypertensive agent, is infrequently used these days due to side effects such as postural hypotension and problem of withdrawal-related rebound hypertension. It also cases troublesome sedation. Direct vasodilators such as hydralazine and minoxidil are effective, but some of their side effects (such as tachycardia, headache, and retention of sodium and water) may make it difficult to use them in modern day treatment of hypertension. Racemic forms of calcium channel blockers and beta-blockers are presently available. However, long-term studies regarding their efficacy and safety are not available.

Follow-up and Other Treatment

After initiation of therapy the patient should be closely monitored for the efficacy and look out for side effects. The blood pressure must be checked every week at clinic or home. Other risk factors should be monitored. The dose of the agents can be increased or second or more drugs can be added to control the blood pressure. Once the blood pressure is controlled the frequency of check ups can be increased to once or 3 months.

Low dose aspirin is prescribed to all hypertensives with cardiovascular disease or stroke (secondary prevention). Aspirin is also advocated for those >50 years, those with renal failure and those at high risk for cardiac disease, those with cardiovascular, cerebrovascular or peripheral vascular disease with LDL cholesterol more than 100 should be given a statin.

Heart Failure

Heart failure (HF) does not mean the heart has stopped working. Rather, it means that the heart's pumping power is weaker than normal. Heart failure can be defined as the inability of the heart or a chamber of heart to deliver enough blood according to the requirements of the body. It can be failure of the right side or the left side of the heart or together as CCF. In left side, it can be left ventricular failure or left atrial failure. Apart from diseased valves myocardial disease is the main cause of heart failure. There is low cardiac output leading to congestion in the chamber and organs upstream: In left heart failure there will be pulmonary edema and in right heart failure (RHF) there will be congestion of liver, and edema of feet. This is also referred to as backward failure. The resulting signs and symptoms of low cardiac output are called forward failure. The normal cardiac index (cardiac output per meter square of body surface area) is 2.4–4.0 L/min/m^2. In heart failure it can decrease to or less than 1l/min/m^2. There can be high output with cardiac index up to 10l/min/m^2 but symptoms of heart failure in conditions like severe anemia, hyperthyroidism, sepsis, beriberi and large arteriovenous shunts.

Epidemiology

HF is the commonest cause for admission in elderly with more than 550,000 new cases diagnosed and 200,000 deaths annually in USA. As IHD and hypertension is being treated earlier these patients live longer and develop HF later on. The incidence of HF doubles every decade after age 45 years and carries a poor prognosis. In the Framingham study the 5-year mortality for men was 62 percent and 42 percent for women.

Causes

1. Left ventricular systolic dysfunction can be due to coronary artery disease, hypertension, mitral valve disease or aortic

valve disease, cardiomyopathy or myocarditis, drugs and T or AF. These cause low output. Anemia, hyperthyroidism and arteriovenous shunt, beriberi and Paget's disease cause high output HF

2. Left atrial failure can occur in mitral stenosis, left atrial myxoma, LV function remains normal
3. Right-sided failure can be due to pulmonary stenosis, tricuspid stenosis or tricuspid regurgitation, pulmonary stenosis, constrictive pericarditis and pulmonary hypertension. The last can be either primary or secondary to left side disease. Constrictive pericarditis causes HF due to reduced filling of RV.

Pathophysiology

Cardiac output depends on heart rate and stroke volume (the volume of blood ejected in each cardiac cycle). One mechanism of compensating for heart failure is increasing heart rate. But beyond 170–180 beats per minute this leaves less diastolic filling time and ultimately output falls. Resting heart rates of over 100 beats per minute is a finding of heart failure and is of bad prognostic significance. Stroke volume is dependent on three factors: Preload, afterload and contractility of heart. "Preload": For the heart to pump blood it must be filled well with blood. Filling blood in heart cavity stretches the cardiac muscle fibers. This filling of heart with blood or length of the muscle fibers before contraction for forward pumping is called the preload. To some extent the pumping is directly related to the amount of blood filled. If there is less blood in heart it will stretch less and obviously pump less forward. This follows the Starling's law described over a century ago: Muscle tension developed is proportional to its stretching (length) within physiological limits.

Afterload: This is the pressure in aorta or pulmonary artery which the heart has to overcome to pump blood forward.
Contractility: Cardiac output is increased by increasing the force of contraction of heart muscles when preload and afterload are constant. Contractility depends on the action of myofibrils. In the cardiac muscle cell this is initiated by the interaction of

intracellular calcium with the contractile protein. Increased calcium influx upon initiation leads to increased contraction (as digitalis or catecholamine) and calcium efflux causes relaxation as with calcium channel blocking drugs and beta-blockers. An increase in contractility leads to a shift of the ventricular function curve to left causing increased output at the same preload.

Cardiac function curve in diagram illustrating the Frank-Starling law of the heart, the Y-axis often describes the stroke volume, stroke work, or cardiac output. The X-axis often describes end-diastolic volume, right atrial pressure, or pulmonary capillary wedge pressure or preload, Frank-Starling curve shows (Fig. 3.1) separate lines, each roughly the same shape, one on top of each other, to illustrate that shifts on the

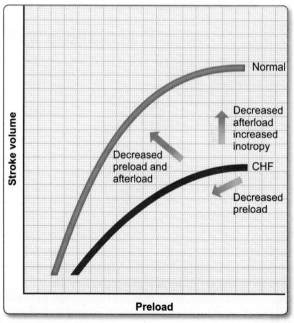

Fig. 3.1: Frank-Starling curve

same line indicate a change in preload, while shifts from one line to another indicate a change in contractility or congestive heart failure (CHF).

If afterload increases the heart muscles stretch and then over time hypertrophy just as muscular training (exercise, weight lifting) increases muscle mass. But beyond a limit the heart fails to work adequately. When conditions for heart failure exist, the body compensates by retaining salt and water and thereby increasing the blood volume. This increases the preload whereby the muscle fibers are stretched and they produce more tension or force and so cardiac output will increase. But beyond some limit (pulmonary wedge pressure > 25 mmHg) the oncotic pressure of the diluted blood is decreased and fluid extravasates from the blood into extravascular compartment causing interstitial edema. If the fibers are stretched too much it fails and cardiac output decreases; this is cardiac failure.

Ejection fraction is a common measure of systolic function. It is the proportion of blood ejected by the ventricle during systole. Hence, it is the percentage of ratio of the volume of blood at the end of systole and at the end of diastole. This can be measured on echocardiogram, angiogram or radionuclide studies.

Neurohormonal Response to Low Cardiac Output

Low cardiac output results in compensatory response form rennin-angiotensin system and adrenergic nervous system. The main goal is to maintain adequate blood flow to vital organs, especially kidneys. Heart failure with less renal blood flow activates the renal angiotensin-aldosterone system resulting in sodium and water retention in the body, increased blood volume, causing increased preload and increasing the cardiac output. Heart failure also actives the sympathetic system with release of adrenergic hormones which increase the heart rate and contractility of heart thereby increasing the cardiac output. The end result of these is increased output at the cost of pulmonary congestion, peripheral edema and increased afterload. Moreover increased LV volume causes increased

wall tension and oxygen demand. In long run this results in LV hypertrophy. In dilated cardiomyopathy as hypertrophy cannot occur failure worsens. The neurohormones on sustained exposure are toxic to heart.

Symptoms

The symptoms depend on whether the left or right side of heart is involved, the etiology and the severity of damage. The earliest sign and often missed is fatigue, and exhaustion even after minor tasks. This can be both in RHF and LHF. In LHF there will be progressive breathlessness on lesser and lesser exertion, orthopnea, paroxysmal nocturnal dyspnea, frank pulmonary edema, dry nocturnal cough, nocturia, giddiness, syncope. In right ventricular failure (RVF) there will be swelling of feet, face and later ascites. Liver congestion can cause pain in right hypochondrium especially on exertion, nausea and anorexia, weight loss and cachexia.

Some symptoms can be seen after treatment like weakness due to hypokalemia (thiazide diuretics), nausea and anorexia (digoxin), postural hypotension (diuretics and all afterload reducing agents), dry nocturnal cough (ACE inhibitors), headache (nitrates).

Signs

Resting tachycardia is a sign of cardiac decompensation and also of poor prognosis. Low blood pressure with low pulse pressure is seen due to decreased cardiac output. The exceptions are mitral and aortic regurgitation (wide pulse pressure).

Jugular veins: It is recorded with patient at 45° angle to the bed. At the sternal angle or angle of Lewis the jugular venous pressure (JVP) is 5 cm above the RA. So a jugular vein column seen 3 cm above this means the RA pressure is 8 cm of H_2O. If the venous column is above this it is considered high. In severe failure the top level may not be seen with patient sitting upright and with low CVP the patient has to be flat to visualize the pulse. A high JVP means RVF except in superior vena cava (SVC) obstruction where no pulsations will be visible (Fig. 3.2).

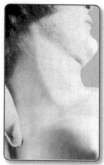

Abdominal jugular reflux (hepatojugular reflux): A pressure on abdomen in peri-umbilical area causes a rise in jugular venous column of about 3 cm normally. In heart failure it rises to much above this level and is also sustained. Normally considered as a sign of RHF, it is also found in LHF due to high pulmonary wedge pressure and RA pressure. It is also seen in tricuspid regurgitation.

Jugular venous pulse has two waves: 'a' wave due to atrial contraction and 'v' wave due to ventricular contraction.

Fig. 3.2: Raised JVP

To see the pulse the patient is positioned in such a way that the pulsations are seen through sternomastoid muscle in neck and simultaneously palpate the brachial pulse to time the ventricular systole. The 'a' wave will be before the brachial pulse and 'v' wave after. A big 'v' wave occurs in tricuspid regurgitation.

Edema is seen on feet and progressively upwards in CHF (Fig. 3.3). Face may also be puffy. Any dependent part like the scrotum, hands will also have edema. Ascites can also occur in RHF.

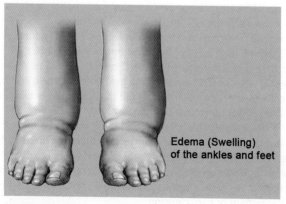

Edema (Swelling) of the ankles and feet

Fig. 3.3: Pedal edema

Examination of Chest

Cheyne-Stokes breathing which is seen primarily in brain disease is also seen in advanced heart failure. Barrel chest of smokers with chronic bronchitis is observed in cor pulmonale. RHF can also occur in kyphoscoliosis. Pleural effusion is usually bilateral or on right usually if unilateral in HF. It can result in reduced breath sounds on that side especially in bases. Pulmonary congestion is reflected by crepitations heard at the end of inspiration initially in bases and in advanced stages all over the chest. The mechanism is the closure of alveoli due to congested interstitial paces of lungs in expiration and an increased inspiratory effort causes these alveoli to pop open at the end of inspiration. Rhonchi and audible wheeze will accompany crepitations in CHF and will be more marked in cases of cor pulmonale due to chronic bronchitis.

Examination of Heart

Apical Impulse

The apical impulse is felt at the point of maximum impulse (PMI) usually in 5th intercostal space in midclavicular line in supine position. It is localized to 2 cm area and tapping in quality. In LVH the apical impulse is forceful. In systolic dysfunction, LV volume overload and dilatation it is shifted towards anterior axillary line and the apex beat is also enlarged so that it is felt in a wider area of 1–2 intercostal spaces. In volume overload the apex beat is diffuse and rocking in nature. The left parasternal region will have a heave in RV volume overload and it will be sustained in RV pressure overload. In AS there will be double impact apex beat. In emphysema the heart is vertical and has clockwise rotation so the PMI is felt in subxiphoid region and is due to RVH due to cor pulmonale.

Thrill is a palpable murmur and is felt in same area as the murmur is heard when the murmur is louder than grade III /VI. Percussion will reveal enlargement of heart when the dullness extends beyond midclavicular line in 5th intercostal space and the pulmonary area will be dull if there is pulmonary artery enlargement or hypertension.

Heart Sounds

S_1 and S_2 are usually normal but may be depressed in advanced heart failure. S_1 may be load in MS or absent in MR and in AF, while P_2 is loud in pulmonary hypertension and A_2 is absent in calcified aortic value. S_3 = big flabby ventricle (volume overload) S_3 is a soft sound low pitched sound best heard with the bell in 3rd or 4th space with patient rolled to left. It is due to rapid ventricular filling and a dilated and complaint ventricle. Best example is cardiomyopathy. It also carries a bad prognosis. When associated with tachycardia is called S_3 gallop. S_4 = stiff noncomplaint LV (afterload) occurs at the end of diastole due to contraction of atria forcing blood into a stiff ventricle as in hypertension, LVH, ischemia, infiltrative diseases. It will be therefore absent when the atrial kick is lost as in atrial fibrillation, AV block, ventricular or nodal rhythm and ventricular pacing. When associated with tachycardia three sounds are like a galloping horse and so are called S_3 or S_4 gallop. If it is not possible to distinguish between S_3 and S_4 with tachycardia it is called summation gallop.

Murmurs

These may point to the etiology of heart failure like a loud systolic murmur of MR or AS; a soft systolic murmur of papillary muscle dysfunction causing mild MR. Murmurs may become soft due to heart failure itself.

Investigations

Laboratory Investigations

All patients should routinely have CBC, urinalysis, renal function tests including electrolytes, liver function tests, blood sugar, thyroid function tests especially if there is AF or in elderly. X-ray chest and ECG are a must. Depending on the etiology of HF, X-ray will show cardiomegaly and prominent vascular markings in LVF, with an appearance of bats wings in frank pulmonary edema. ECG will show LVH or RVH, LA or RA enlargement, AF, VPCs, etc.

Echocardiography

This is the most useful test. It will tell about the heart function as also about the etiology of HF. It will also define regional wall motion abnormalities in ischemic heart disease. Wall motion abnormality like hypokinesia, akinesia or dyskinesia suggests coronary heart disease while global hypokinesia implies cardiomyopathy.

Radionuclide angiogram or MUGA scan is helpful when echocardiography is difficult as in obese patient or in emphysema. Radioisotopes labeled red cells are injected and the scanning is done in systole and diastole to give the LVEF.

Brain natriuretic peptide (BNP) first isolated form brain and therefore so named, BNP is released by stretched myocytes. When there is heart failure, LV volume increases and therefore myocytes are stretched and they release BNP. It is increased in HF due to systolic and diastolic dysfunction. A normal level excludes heart failure and it is useful to distinguish whether the cause of dyspnea is cardiac or respiratory. A level above 100 pg/mL usually indicated HF. Marked elevation of BNP above 130 pg/mL suggests poor prognosis and a higher risk of sudden death. BNP increases with age and is higher in women. A high BNP at the time of discharge is associated with higher readmission rate and needs aggressive treatment. BNP release is a counter regulatory response to the actions of sympathetic and rennin angiotensin-aldosterone systems in short term it does not boost cardiac output, in long term it increases natriuresis, blocks sympathetic and rennin-angiotensin-aldosterone system, causes arterial and venodilatation.

Endomyocardial Biopsy

This required in few patients to establish a diagnosis of HF. It is used to diagnose viral, infiltrative cardiomyopathy.

Treatment of Heart Failure

Nonpharmacologic Treatment

A patient with HF should have complete bed rest to reduce cardiac work. Once patient is better he is encouraged to do all activities gradually. Salt restriction is very useful as also fluid restriction to the tune of about 1000 mL per day in congested patients abstinence from alcohol is essential for alcoholic cardiomyopathy and thiamine is given.

Pharmacologic Treatment
Beta Adrenergic Blockade
A failing heart needs some β adrenergic support. But increasing levels of circulating catecholamines and decreasing number of myocardial receptors is toxic. Beta adrenergic blockade is therefore helpful and is the most important treatment for HF. Initially they are started at 1/16 to 1/8 of the target dose and titrated up gradually every 2–3 weeks. A heart rate of 60/min means there is good beta-blockade. Temporary worsening of symptoms may occur initially. Be careful to start this if resting heart rate is less than 60/min or systolic blood pressure is less than 100 mmHg. LVEF increases after β blockade, in some up to 15 percent. Maximum benefit is for those whose LVEF increases most. It is useful in all grades of HF I-IV. Long-acting metoprolol is started in a dose of 12.5 mg and up titrated to 50–200 mg/day. Carvidilol is started as 3.125 mg twice a day and increased to 25–50 mg/day. There is no clear cut benefit of one over the other, but carvedilol may be useful in class IV HF. Atenolol may be started at 12.5 mg/day. Nebivolol and bisoprolol have also been used with similar effects. In patients with bronchospasm metoprolol or nebivolol may be useful.

Angiotensin Converting Enzyme Inhibitors
These form the second cornerstone of therapy for HF. They block conversion of angiotensin I to angiotensin II which is powerful vasoconstrictor thereby causing vasodilatation and reduction of afterload. This increases cardiac output without increasing myocardial work (one of the rare occasions in life where you get something without any effort!). They are indicated in all grades of HF including asymptomatic LV dysfunction (LVEF <40%). It is class effect. Initial trials were with captopril or enalapril. Recent HOPE trail showed that they prevent HF in 25 percent and the greatest benefit was in those with hypertension. The

most common side effect is a dry hacking cough more at night which occurs in up to 15 percent cases and is not relived by cough suppressants. It is due to potentiation of bradykinin. Oral iron is effective for it sometimes If not relived then patient can be shifted to angiotensin receptor blocker (ARB). Second side effect is angioedema. ACE inhibitors are contraindicated in pregnancy due to fetal abnormalities and neonatal morbidity and mortality.

It can increase creatinine in patient of renal artery stenosis (RAS). So check creatinine a couple of days after starting ACE inhibitor and if it rises by 0.3 mg/dL or more, stop the drug and investigate for RAS. Hyperkalemia is another problem if there is renal dysfunction, or potassium sparing diuretics or potassium supplements are given. Elevated creatinine above 2.5–3 mg/dL is a contraindication to use of ACE inhibitors. Hypotension is another side effect which is common if serum sodium is less than 140 mg/dL, when patient is dry or on diuretics. It can be avoided by giving a diuretic holiday for a couple of days when starting ACR inhibitors. If hypotension occurs, diuretics can be stopped and ACE inhibitors can be restarted with a smaller dose.

Angiotensin receptor blocker (ARB) losartan, valsartan, irbesartan, candesartan and telmisartan are all equally effective in HF as ACE inhibitors. Adding valsartan to ACE inhibitor may be good especially if hypertensive. But Val-HeFT trial found the triple combination of BB, ACE inhibitors and ARB is not well-tolerated.

Afterload Reduction with Other Drugs

Hydralazine at a high dose of 300 mg/day in four divided doses is useful. It can be combined with isosorbide 160 mg/day. But side effects are very common and very few patients can continue this high dose. Smaller doses than this are possibly not beneficial.

Aldosterone Antagonists

Spironolactone and eplerenone improve symptoms and survival in HF class III and IV (RALES trial). Thirty-five percent reduction in rehospitalization was reported possibly due to less myocardial and vascular fibrosis. Side effects are gynecomastia, hyperkalemia especially in renal dysfunction.

Inotropic Therapy

Digoxin is helpful in most patients with advanced symptoms. Indeed stopping digoxin while continuing ACE inhibitors worsened symptoms. The DIG trial showed that it improved symptoms, reduced hospitalization for HF, but did not increase mortality. Thus, it is now recommended when ACE inhibitors, BB, diuretics do not control symptoms. It may be given at 0.125 dose to prevent side effects as patients with HF may be elderly or have hepatic or renal dysfunction all of which increase side effects. Noncardiac toxic symptoms are visual changes, nausea or anorexia. Side effects

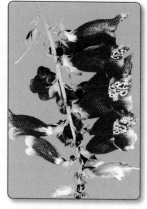

Fig. 3.4: Digitalis purpurea plant whose extract first helped in heart failure

are common when associated with hypokalemia. Check blood digitalis and potassium levels. Bradycardia, ventricular ectopy especially ventricular bigeminy, heart blocks are common cardiac side effects (Fig. 3.4).

Dobutamine Infusion

This is useful in acute decompensated HF with hypotension especially with renal dysfunction with diuretics. It reverses hemodynamic abnormalities: Pulmonary wedge pressure falls and cardiac output increases. It does not improve survival, hospital stay or readmission. It is useful for relief of symptoms. At a dose of 408 µg/kg/min it reduces systemic and pulmonary vascular resistance and improves cardiac output without raising heart rate or myocardial oxygen demand. Urine output is improves. In end stage HF it can be given at home for 6 hours 4 times a week.

Milrinone is another drug with similar effects with less effect on heart rate and ventricular ectopy.

Dopamine increases output but is accompanied by detrimental tachycardia. There is no documented 'renal dose' effect on urine output. It should not be used if dobutamine is available.

Preload Reduction
Diuretics

Pulmonary or systemic congestion is improved with diuretics. It improves cardiac output initially by pushing on the flat part of ventricular function curve. Later it moves patent down and reduced cardiac output. It does not improve survival but helps symptoms. Once congestion is removed and other drugs are in place it can be withdrawn. Lop diuretics like furosemide or torsemide are used but the effectiveness is impaired due to reduced absorption upto 70 percent, spanchnic edema, liver failure and hypotension causing less drug delivery to the nephrons. It can be given in repeated doses or in an infusion to overcome this diuretic resistance: 40 mg loading dose and then 10–40 mg/hour. Maximum dose is 160–200 mg/day for furosemide intravenous and twice that orally in normal renal function, higher in renal failure. With higher doses needed in pulmonary edema there can be tinnitus. Torsemide has similar actions as furosemide but has longer half-life and better oral bioavailability even in presence of splanchnic congestion. Intravenously there is no difference between both. It can be effectively given in two doses: For furosemide 4 hours apart and for torsemide 6 hours apart in morning and noon. It can be combined with thiazide HCTZ 100–200 mg/day or metallozone. Occasional patient will respond to spironolactone. Dose is 50–200 mg/day. It may be a couple of weeks before diuresis begins. 50 mg spironolactone per day spares potassium and increases magnesium by 13 percent side effect is hypokalemia found equally with loop diuretics as with thiazides. Secondly thiamine deficiency occurs as diuretics wash out thiamine.

Nesiritide: Human recombinant brain natriuretic peptide is evadible for use in acute pulmonary edema and those not responding to other treatment. It has to be given intravenously and it effectively reduced pulmonary wedge pressure. However curiously symptoms may not subside.

Vasopressin receptor blockers—are under trail for HF.

Other Therapy for Heart Failure

Biventricular pacing resynchronization therapy is useful for HF with LBBB with wide QRS > 130 m/sec. By pacing both sides of ventricle the function improve and prevents sudden cardiac death. MR tends to improve. However, the pacemaker is very expensive.

Ultrafiltration: This has shown promise for HF. It can reduce water to the tune of 1–2 L/hour.

Implantable Defibrillator

Patient of HF die of sudden cardiac death due to ventricular fibrillation. This has been reduced in patients implanted with this device which shocks the heart whenever the VT occurs. The device is very expensive.

Surgery

Ventricular remodeling and cardiac transplant are two surgical alternatives.

Rheumatic Fever

Incidence

Rheumatic fever (RF) is rare these days in developed countries, although complacency in its control there has produced a resurgence in many parts of USA and the UK. Indian statistics are not complete; it is estimated that there are more than 1 million patients with rheumatic heart disease in India. Conservative estimates put the incidence of acute RF at 50,000 new cases per year. A special feature of this disease in India is the early onset of symptomatic valvular disease in children; a few of these can be truly malignant in their clinical course (Juvenile rheumatic heart disease).

The disease is common in childhood and adolescence, and is rare in infants and in old age and attacks the poor, especially those living in damp, dirty, and unhygienic surroundings. Its incidence parallels that of streptococcal tonsillitis. Although rare in adults, it presents with more severe joint disease in them. The saying is "it licks the joint but bites the heart in children and licks the heart and bites the joint in older patients"; however this may not always be correct. Figure 4.1 gives the natural history of RF.

Genetics

Genetic factors have been implicated in the pathogenesis and it is not infrequent to find multiple cases in one family. The present data support the hypothesis of a rheumatic fever gene within or near the HLA complex. Patients with RF may have an abnormal immunological response both at the humoral and cellular levels to streptococcal antigens cross-reactive with mammalian tissue. This abnormal response is likely to be genetically programmed.

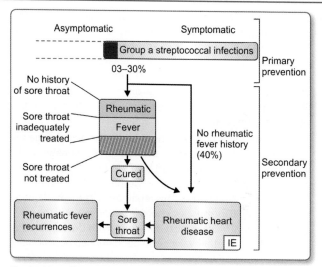

Fig. 4.1: Natural history of rheumatic fever

Etiopathogenesis

There is, as yet, no proof of an infective agent causing RF, though it is nearly always preceded by streptococcal sore throat, the latent interval being 10–20 days.

Rheumatic fever is the result of an abnormal immune response to the products of hemolytic streptococcal infection in a sensitized individual. It is possible that some of the antibodies to antigens present on the streptococcal cell wall may cross-react with myofibrils in the heart, thereby setting up pancarditis.

Pathology

Fulminating attacks which end fatally show only non-specific changes like the Arthus phenomenon, seen in many other acute infections. Edema, fragmentation of collagen, leukocyte infiltration, hyperemia and capillary hemorrhage are seen in synovial membranes of the larger joints, pericardium, myocardium, endocardium, the pleura and the lungs.

The classical rheumatic lesion, however, is proliferative. This occurs later, the best example being the Aschoff nodule. The subcutaneous nodule is another example. A necrotic collagenous center is surrounded by large multinucleated reticuloendothelial cells, along with lymphocytes and plasma cells. This is seen in the myocardium near blood vessels. Fibroblastic proliferation is usual. Rarely panarteritis of many viscera may be seen.

A true valvulitis occurs in the heart. In the acute stage the valve is edematous, and soon shows signs of damage to the area of maximum apposition just below its free edge. Small pink nodules may be seen at this stage. The inflamed valves later get fibrosed and fusion occurs. This repair process might damage the valves, papillary muscles, chordae tendineae, and the valve rings. The mitral valve is most damaged, with the aortic valve next in order; the other valves also get damaged occasionally.

Clinical Features

Rheumatic fever is a systemic disease with varied clinical presentations (Fig. 4.2). Although subclinical attacks may not have significant joint involvement, clinical presentation without joint involvement is very rare.

Arthritis: This is usually polyarthritis, sometimes flitting from joint to joint (migratory), affecting the larger joints more than the smaller ones. Swelling, redness and tenderness are the common findings and occasionally joint effusions. Vague pain in the joints may not be a feature of this disease. Joint manifestations are more prominent in adults. History of sore throat 2–4 weeks prior to the joint involvement may be obtained in some people.

Skin lesions: The classical erythema marginatum—large erythematous lesions with prominent margins slightly raised—are seen more often in white people and is rare in Indians. The red margins take longer to fade and so the lesions sometimes look like red rings.

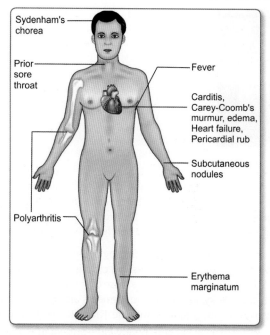

Fig. 4.2: Clinical features of the rheumatic fever

Subcutaneous nodules: These are painless, roundish, firm lumps overlaid by normal looking skin (Fig. 4.3). They range from a few millimeters to 1.5 cm in diameter, and are localized over bony prominences like the elbow, shin and spine. If carefully looked for, these are not as rare as reported. They sometimes last longer than a month.

Carditis: This is the single most important lesion. It presents with breathlessness, chest pain of pericardial type, and palpitations due to tachycardia. Cardiac enlargement with heart murmurs is not uncommon. The mitral valve being the most common valve involved, a soft middiastolic murmur due to thickening of the mitral valve, the Carey-Coombs murmur, is the classical picture; in practice, a soft systolic murmur is more common. Pericardial rub may be heard at some stage in the disease.

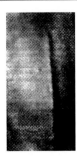

Fig. 4.3: Subcutaneous nodules

Severe carditis with mitral and aortic valve leaks may result in heart failure; heart failure may also be due to myocarditis. The latter may present with heart blocks and syncope. A fulminant course is not uncommon in the tropics where the disease progresses to heart failure and death in a very short time.

Rheumatic chorea: Described first by Sydenham, this clumsy movement of the limb muscles in a child is rarely a feature of acute RF. It is usually seen after a lapse of 4–6 weeks, during the cold stage. Jerky, involuntary movements are the feature and they usually subside after sometime. The child may be thought of as being restless or inattentive in school.

Fever: This is usually a feature during the acute phase. Pleurisy, pneumonia, and occasionally pleural effusion may also be seen but are rare.

Modified Duckett-Jones criteria: The clinical features of this disease have been grouped into major and minor criteria by Duckett-Jones; these have been revised by the American Heart Association. A diagnosis of rheumatic fever is likely when two major criteria are present or when one major criterion is seen along with two minor ones, along with evidence of past streptococcal infection (Table 4.1).

Investigations

Routine blood counts and erythrocyte sedimentation rate (ESR) are nonspecific but are useful for follow up. Throat cultures for

Table 4.1: Jones criteria (revised by American heart association, 1984)

Major		Minor
	Clinical	
Carditis		Fever
Polyarthritis		Arthralgia
Chorea		Postrheumatic fever or rheumatic heart disease
Erythema marginatum		
Subcutaneous nodules		
	Laboratory	
		Elevated ESR
		CRP positive
		Leukocytosis
		Prolonged PR interval
	Plus	

Supporting evidence of preceding streptococcal infection (increased ASO or other streptococcal antibodies; positive throat culture for group A streptococcus; recent scarlet fever).

streptococci are helpful. Anti-streptolysin O (ASO) titers are useful if there is a rising titer or, in its absence, levels above 200 units. In many patients this may be normal.

ECG evidence of carditis is not infrequent. Prolonged PR interval, varying grades of heart block and occasionally repolarization changes (ST-T changes) may suggest pericardial or myocardial involvement. Echocardiography may help to diagnose cardiomegaly and/or pericardial effusion. Valve damage may also be seen (Table 4.2).

Management

Supportive therapy: Bed rest is important and activity should be curtailed until the ESR comes to normal. Heart failure when

Table 4.2: Work-up in a case of acute rheumatic fever

Blood	CBC (leukocytosis), ESR (raised), C-reactive protein (raised)
	ASO titer (raised > 200 units)
Throat	Throat swab for β-hemolytic streptococci.
Chest X-ray	Cardiomegaly
ECG	Increased PR interval (I degree heart block, rarely II degree heart block)
	If pericarditis—Low voltage, T wave inversion
2D-echo	For valve abnormality and cardiomegaly

Table 4.3: Differential diagnosis

1. Rheumatoid arthritis: Small joints are involved, not migratory; older age group is affected, females more often; deformities of joints are seen, small muscle wasting may be seen, and the serology is diagnostic.

2. Osteoarthritis: Older age, single joint involvement, and effusion are more common; Heberden's nodes may be seen in the fingers; serology is negative.

3. Gouty arthritis: Usually the great toe is affected but it could be polyarthritic; tophi may be seen. Older men are affected, uric acid levels are high and the clinical presentation is very typical.

4. Systemic lupus erythematosus: The clinical picture and laboratory tests should distinguish it.

5. Lyme disease: Usually seen in the West, it presents with annular erythematous skin rashes, knee joint pain, fever, heart blocks and similar serological features.

6. Fibrositis: Muscular rheumatism is a vague syndrome of adults where minor aches and pains mostly reflect their mild depressive illness. The clinical picture is typical and the joint involvement is only an arthralgia.

7. Septic arthritis: In children this should be easy to distinguish as the clinical presentation is more dramatic with signs of systemic infection, and the joint fluid will grow the organism.

8. TB joints: Joint signs are classical, and systemic manifestations may be seen. A single joint is involved except in the spine.

9. Adverse drug reaction: Arthralgia is a common feature of allergy seen with many drugs. Multiple joints may be affected and the skin lesions and history will be diagnostic.

present needs attention. If the fulminant disease progresses to valve damage, rarely surgery may be needed on an urgent basis. Heart blocks are usually transient and rarely need pacing.

Salicylates: Aspirin in large doses (60 mg/kg body weight in six divided doses) is the drug of choice. In adults double this dose can be given. This should be continued till the ESR comes down and then tapered off. Nausea, tinnitus, vomiting, deafness, and rarely tachypnea and acidosis may be the side effects. Reye's syndrome precludes its use in small children.

Steroids: These are more useful in symptom relief especially in severe cases, although there is no long-term advantage compared to aspirin. Prednisolone in doses of 0.25 mg/Kg body weight in divided doses is given until the ESR comes to normal and then tapered off over 3–4 weeks.

Antibiotics: To treat the streptococcal infection an initial dose of 1,200,000 units of benzathine penicillin should be given, initially once a week for three weeks and then monthly for the Ist year. Long-term prophylaxis is still debated. Benzathine penicillin 1,200,000 units monthly or three weekly, or oral phenoxymethyl penicillin 500 mg daily may be continued until the age of 40 years. Benzathine penicillin once in 2 weeks may give better results than the monthly dose. In community studies long-term penicillin has been shown to reduce the incidence of streptococcal reinfection but in individuals there is no proof of that. In penicillin-sensitive individuals erythromycin or sulfadiazine are preferred (Table 4.3).

Long-term Care

These patients need follow-up on a regular basis to rule out cardiac valvular involvement, preferably by echocardiography. When present, its management with drugs or surgery may be required. Carditis is seen usually within weeks of the onset but may rarely be seen for the first time after the 4th week. Recurrence of RF is very common and must be prevented by antibiotic prophylaxis and also by change in the environment of the patient.

Valvular Heart Disease

Herein we will look into the acquired valvular heart disease. The commonest cause is rheumatic fever (RF) in India. The second is degenerative and third sclerotic. Rheumatic heart disease (RHD) is a common cause of cardiac morbidity and mortality in India. Studies have shown prevalence rates to range from 25 to 60 percent (average 40%) of all patients hospitalized for heart disease. The prevalence amongst school children varies from 1.8/1000 to 11/1000, with a national average of 6/1000. Epidemiological studies show a prevalence rate of upto 5.1 per 1000 in the rural population and 1.6 per 1000 in the urban population.

Clinical Pattern of Valvular Involvement

The clinical pattern of valve involvement in RHD reported from various centers in India shows a predominant mitral valve involvement, followed by combined mitral and aortic valve disease, with isolated aortic valve disease being very uncommon. Rheumatic tricuspid valve disease does not occur in isolation. As functional tricuspid regurgitation it commonly accompanies mitral stenosis with pulmonary arterial hypertension. Clinical evidence of tricuspid regurgitation (trivial to severe; functional or organic) is noted in 40 percent of patients with mitral valve disease. Tricuspid stenosis occurs invariably in accompaniment with mitral stenosis. Amongst the mitral valve lesions, isolated mitral stenosis or dominant mitral stenosis with trivial or mild mitral regurgitation occurs frequently. Isolated mitral regurgitation is uncommon. Isolated aortic valve disease consists predominantly of aortic regurgitation.

Mitral Stenosis

Mitral stenosis (MS) is almost synonymous with rheumatic heart disease (RHD). It may be associated with aortic valve diseases but isolated aortic valve disease is usually not due to RHD. Rheumatic fever is caused by antigenic reaction to streptococcal throat infection. The antibodies attack cardiac vales, mitral being the commonest. The valve becomes thickened and later calcified and narrowed. It may also fail to coapt causing regurgitation. In India and in other developing countries an attack of RF is aggressive and is quickly followed by valvular heart disease in a matter of few years, say the RF occurs in teens and the mitral stenosis is detected in late teens or early twenties. In developed world it takes decades to manifest so that the RF in childhood is followed by valvular heart disease in 4th or 5th decade. The pattern of RHD in India shows several differences from that reported in the West. Severe symptomatic RHD occurring in the younger age group (below 20 years of age) is far more frequent here. The average age of a patient with RHD in UK was 37 years which is at least 15 years more than the average age of the Indian patient. The rheumatic calendar in India is thus markedly advanced, with florid clinical manifestations of crippling valvular lesions occurring at a much younger age. This feature was originally noted in patients of mitral stenosis and was described as 'juvenile mitral stenosis' but has subsequently been noted in the entire spectrum of RHD. Male preponderance has been noted by most investigators from India. This is in contradiction to the female preponderance noted in mitral stenosis in the West.

Pathophysiology

In rheumatic fever there is streptococcal infection of the throat. The antibodies produced by the body to fight that cross reacts with some substance of the cardiac valves. There is resulting inflammation of the cardiac valve. The inflamed valve may not close properly and may cause temporary regurgitation. The inflammation resolves with joining and fibrosis of the commissures of the valve resulting in short thick, rigid cusps with narrow valve opening. This is stenosis of the valve. This may also involve a valve with fixed aperture and regurgitation. There can be calcification also on the valves. These changes may take decades to occur.

Because of MS or MR there is increased LA pressure. This is reflected in increased pressure in pulmonary veins and capillaries. There is increased interstitial fluid causing stiff lungs. MS is a disease of the lungs in this sense. It may cause pulmonary edema. If the pulmonary capillary pressure exceeds 25 mmHg and the resulting transudation cannot be cleared by the lymphatics, acute pulmonary edema develops. The engorged pulmonary capillaries may rupture causing hemoptysis which is a hallmark of MS. As a compensatory measure pulmonary artery pressure increases and thereby protects lung from flooding. This results in RV overload and failure. This causes RA pressure increase, increased SVC or IVC pressure. Jugular veins will become distended and liver congested and peripheral edema and ascites.

A stenosed valve, enlarged LA and AF all lead to blood stagnation in LA. This causes a clot which can remains in LA or may break up and embolize systemic emboli due to dislodgement of left atrial thrombi may present as cerebrovascular accidents, as embolic occlusion of the peripheral arteries of the limbs, or dramatically as a saddle embolus at the aortic bifurcation. Embolic episodes are far more common in patients who have developed atrial fibrillation. Pulmonary embolism may develop in patients with congestive heart failure.

The striking observations that have been made in Indian studies on *juvenile mitral stenosis* are (1) severe valvular pathology with critically reduced mitral orifice (< 1.0 cm^2) and marked subvalvular and cuspal fusion along with commissural fusion; (2) evidence of severe pulmonary hypertension; (3) low occurrence of valve calcification (< 10%) and (4) uncommon left atrial thrombi and systemic embolization, possibly due to the low incidence of atrial fibrillation. (5) the changes on valves occur within a few months to years rather than decades as seen in Western world.

Symptoms

The time interval between the onset of symptoms of RF and presentation of symptomatic disease is relatively short in

India. Critical mitral stenosis with severe pulmonary arterial hypertension and congestive heart failure may occur within 1–2 years of the initial illness, the interval in some cases being apparently as short as 6 months. Due to MS there is reduced preload for left ventricle resulting in low cardiac output. This manifests as tiredness, fatigue. These symptoms are nonspecific, insidious, and often ignored by patient. The pulmonary congestion causes dyspnea on exertion and "winter bronchitis". When pulmonary hypertension develops they will have edema over feet, right hypochondrial pain due to liver congestion. Hemoptysis is an alarming symptom which usually stops as soon as the relevant veins collapse after the rupture. Hemoptysis may be due to (1) severe pulmonary venous hypertension resulting in hemorrhage from the pulmonary veins (pulmonary apoplexy), (2) pink frothy sputum accompanying pulmonary edema, (3) blood-streaked sputum of bronchitis, (4) rusty sputum of resolving pneumonitis or (5) pulmonary infarction due to pulmonary embolism the enlarged LA causes atrial fibrillation to develop which will result in palpitations. Hoarseness of voice may occur secondary to left recurrent laryngeal nerve paralysis due to compression by LA (Ortner syndrome). Severe pulmonary hypertension may present as chest pain or as fatigue and decreased exercise tolerance due to low cardiac output.

Signs

There is a butterfly like rash on cheek bones in MS. In case of RV failure there will be raised CVP, palpable, tender liver and pedal edema. The pulse is generally normal but in extreme stenosis it is fast and of small volume. It may be regular, or irregular because of associated atrial arrhythmias. The blood pressure is normal or slightly reduced. The S_1 can be felt as a taping ape beat. If there is RV hypertrophy, there is a parasternal heave felt. A loud first heart sound due to closure of the diseased mitral valve with rapid apposition of leaflets which are well-separated at end-diastole, is an important auscultatory sign of mitral stenosis. A low-intensity first heart sound suggests calcification of the mitral valve or dominant associated mitral or aortic regurgitation. The second heart sound is usually normally split with an accentuated pulmonary component reflecting pulmonary arterial hypertension. An important auscultatory feature is the mitral opening snap (os). This sharp and snappy sound, which occurs 30–100 msec after the second heart sound, is due to elevated left atrial pressure which sharply forces open the mitral valve during diastole. As the mitral stenosis increases in severity and the left atrial pressure rises, the mitral valve opens earlier and the S_2-os interval narrows. The OS is absent in a calcified or severely fibrotic mitral valve. The A_2-OS distance was the means of judging the severity of MS in preechocardiography era. The flow of blood across the stenosed valve causes a low pitched rumbling murmur due to the small gradient of about 10–15 mmHg usually found in MS. It is best heard at the apex, with the patient rolled to the left side and with the bell of the stethoscope applied lightly on the chest wall. The murmur is accentuated by the atrial contraction just before the closure of MV and forces the blood in LA across the stenosed valve. The duration of the murmur (rather than its loudness) is a useful auscultatory clue to the severity of the stenotic lesion. With severe stenosis (mitral valve area < 1 cm^2) the murmur is characteristically long, loud, and present throughout diastole with presystolic crescendo component marching into the loud first heart sound. The presystolic crescendo of the mitral stenotic murmur is present with regular sinus rhythm or during atrial fibrillation with short diastolic periods, as long as the mitral valve remains flexible. Its absence is suggestive of a rigid or calcified mitral valve or of a very low cardiac output. S_1 becomes soft or inaudible if the valve is calcified or in AF. In a patient suspected to have mitral stenosis but presenting clinically as severe pulmonary arterial hypertension, tricuspid regurgitation and congestive heart failure with adequate decongestion and improved cardiac output following appropriate medical therapy, the 'silent mitral stenosis' may become apparent with the diastolic murmur becoming well audible. Other murmurs that may be noted in association with isolated mitral stenosis are (1) systolic murmur of functional tricuspid regurgitation and

(2) basal decrescendo early diastolic Graham Steell murmur of hypertensive pulmonary regurgitation, both of which are secondary to severe pulmonary arterial hypertension. However, the accompanying tricuspid regurgitation is frequently due to organic involvement of the tricuspid valve in the Indian setting and the early diastolic murmur heard in association with mitral stenosis is commonly due to associated aortic regurgitation rather than due to pulmonary regurgitation.

Investigations

ECG the rhythm is sinus or atrial flutter or AF. There is rightward shift of QRS axis to right due to RVH. There is LA enlargement seen ('P' mitrale) in the form of (1) a widened and bifid, notched or flat-topped 'p' wave in lead V_1. Tall-peaked P waves (P pulmonale) may develop in the presence of severe pulmonary hypertension, though biatrial enlargement is common even in such patients. R wave is taller than S in V_1 and V_2 and deep S in V_5 and V_6 due to RVH.

X-ray: The left atrial enlargement is one of the earliest signs of mitral stenosis. In early stages it may be limited to enlargement of the left atrial appendage causing straightening of the left heart border. In more advanced cases, the left atrium is recognized as a double density within the cardiac silhouette. Left atrial enlargement is best quantified by a barium esophagogram in the lateral view, with posterior deviation of the barium-filled esophagus. With significant left atrial enlargement, the left main bronchus may be elevated. Giant-sized left atria are seen only with associated mitral regurgitation (Figs 5.1A and B).

Evidence of pulmonary venous hypertension with redistribution of blood flow to the upper lobe veins is characteristic. As the severity increases, a generalized haze appears with features of interstitial and alveolar pulmonary edema. Kerley B lines, which are fine, parallel densities in the peripheral lung fields running perpendicular to the pleural surface, most frequently seen in the costophrenic angles, signify severe pulmonary venous hypertension. These lines are due to thickened interlobular septa. Pulmonary hemosiderosis and ossification are rare radiological manifestations of severe pulmonary venous hypertension (Fig. 5.2).

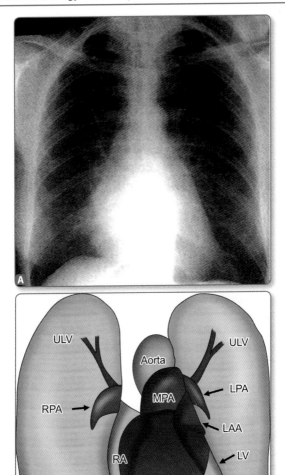

Figs 5.1A and B: X-ray chest in mitral stenosis (MS)
Abbreviations: KL—Kerley lines, LV—left ventricle, RV—right ventricle, RA—right atrium, LAA—left atrial appendage, LPA—left pulmonary artery, MPA—main pulmonary artery, RPA—right pulmonary artery

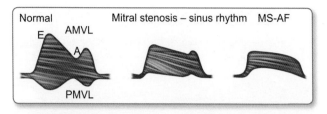

Fig. 5.2: The echocardiogram findings in MS

Pulmonary arterial hypertension with peripheral oligemia may be seen in severe stenosis.

Cardiomegaly results from right ventricular enlargement or a combination of left atrial and right ventricular enlargement with right atrial enlargement contributing only in patients with significant tricuspid regurgitation. Cardiomegaly is present in more than half of Indian patients with mitral stenosis.

Calcification of the mitral valve, the most convincing radiological evidence of a diseased mitral valve, is rare. Calcification of the left atrial wall is an even more uncommon sign and alerts the clinician to the dangers of associated left atrial thrombus and systemic embolism.

Echocardiography is diagnostic and is useful to quantify the stenosis. In M mode it will show flattened, thickened echoes. It may be calcified. In 2-D the valve is seen thickened, deformed and with restricted movements, doming of valve, and calcification. In cross-section, the valve area can be estimated. Doppler can measure the severity from the flow velocity across the valve. The PA will show pulmonary hypertension with Doppler. LA, RV and RV are enlarged. There may be TR due to pulmonary hypertension. Doppler will also reveal if there is associated MR or involvement of AV (Fig. 5.3).

Treatment

The main treatment of MS is opening of the valve either surgically or percutaneously by a balloon catheter. The medical therapy is only to control the symptoms of congestion and the heart rate but is not corrective.

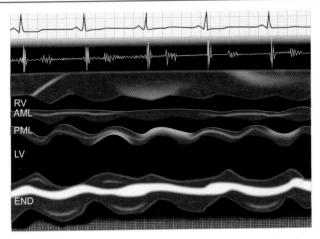

Figs 5.3: Echocardiogram showing loss of M shape of AML in M mode echoes and thickening of MV

Surgery

Mitral stenosis (MS) can be relieved by mitral commissurotomy. The most important thing is the timing of surgery. When patient is symptomatic, has pulmonary hypertension or has had an episode of peripheral embolism surgery is indicated. If done before the valve is calcified, it can be done through the left thoracotomy approach and is called closed mitral valvotomy (CMV) or by open heart operation when it is called open mitral valvotomy (OMV). If the valve is calcified or there is associated MR then the valve has to be replaced by a mechanical or bioprosthetic valve.

Balloon valvotomy can be done if the valve is pliable, there is no calcification or MR. The long-term results of CMV or OMV are better than BMV.

Medical Therapy

If there is congestive heart failure diuretics will help. Digoxin is indicated if there is AF. Beta-blockers can reduce heart rate, increase diastolic filling time for LV and improve symptoms.

Calcium channel blockers like verapamil is indicated in AF. Anticoagulation is indicated if there is a clot on the MV, if there is AF or after MVR with a mechanical valve. The patients need infective endocarditis prophylaxis.

Mitral Regurgitation

Mitral regurgitation (MR) is caused by rheumatic fever (commonest), mitral valve prolapse, ischemic papillary muscle involvement or LV dilatation. Rheumatic MR is often associated with MS and AV involvement also. MR with ischemic heart disease may be acute; in other cases it is chronic.

Pathophysiology

MR causes blood to flow into the low pressure LA during LV systole. During diastole the blood flows back to LV. The LV has to pump more blood so as to maintain blood flow to aorta. So LV dilates. LA receives normal inflow from lungs and in addition the regurgitant flow across the MV. The thin-walled LA therefore gives way and dilates. LV has to pump against a low pressure LA and a high pressure aorta, thereby net afterload is low and LV can eject more forcefully and LVEF is artificially high. After MVR the afterload increases as the LV can no longer dump into low pressure LA. Enlarged LA can lead to AF. Clots in LA usually occur only in AF are commoner in MS.

The net result of MR is similar to MS with pulmonary congestion and later on RV failure. As LVEF is high patient may have a high pulse pressure.

The difference in acute MR is the rapidity of flooding of LA and pulmonary capillaries. There is no time for LA to enlarge so pulmonary edema is rapid.

Symptoms

MR is generally well-tolerated for long due to low afterload. The symptoms are same as in MS: Fatigue, dyspnea, palpitation. Much later RV failure can cause liver congestion and pedal edema. Acute MR occurs with myocardial infarction and papillary muscle dysfunction and presents as florid pulmonary edema.

Signs

The apex beat is shifted downward and outward and is diffuse over more than one intercostal space and is heaving but not sustained (volume overload). S_1 is soft and a S_3 is heard due to rapid filling in diastole. The murmur is holosystolic, extending to S_2 and best audible at apex but radiating to axilla. MR due to papillary muscle dysfunction would be heard best along the sternum as the jet is directed towards the base and may be diamond-shaped crescendo decrescendo due to LV dysfunction. Signs of LV failure like crepitations may be heard over lung bases (Fig. 5.4).

Tests

X-ray chest shows an enlarged cardiac silhouette with LV type of prominence. LA enlargement causes a double contour on right heart border. There will be prominent vascular markings and pulmonary artery shadow may be prominent due to pulmonary hypertension. In pulmonary edema a four wings appearance of confluent shadows radiating from the hilum is seen.

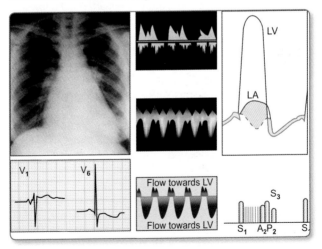

Fig. 5.4: Composite figure showing X-ray, ECG, echocardiogram, pressure tracings and phonocardiogram in MR

ECG shows LVH and LA enlargement (Fig. 5.5).

Echocardiogram is diagnostic and will tell the cause of systolic murmur. It will show the thickened valve of rheumatic MR or the elongated redundant valve leaflets of mitral valve prolapse (MVP). The chorda or papillary muscle may have ruptured. Calcification, associated lesions like MS, AV lesions, vegetations will be seen. LA and LV are enlarged. Doppler and color flow mapping will show the regurgitant jet and its direction and length. LVEF may be high. As it declines after surgery, a LVEF < 50 percent preoperatively is bad. A LV end diastolic volume > 4.5 cm makes for a high risk for surgery (Fig. 5.6).

Treatment

Afterload reduction is useful. ACE inhibitors give symptomatic relief especially in LV failure and reduce LV size. In LVF standard treatment like digoxin, diuretics are also indicated. Definitive treatment is surgery, either repair or replacement.

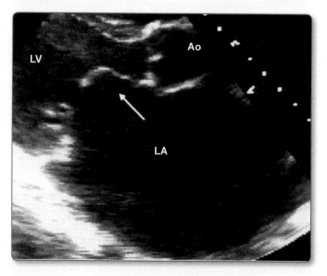

Fig. 5.5: Echocardiogram showing enlarged LA, elbowing of AML

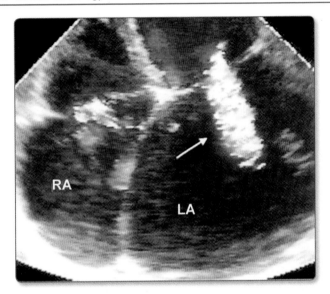

Fig. 5.6: Doppler echocardiogram showing MR jet in LA (arrow)

Surgery: As MR patients remain asymptomatic for years, the timing of surgery is decided by following them with echocardiogram. If LVEF starts declining or LV end diastolic volume increases, surgery is indicated. The risk increases otherwise. MV repair should be done if feasible with replacement only for deformed, calcified valves. Mortality is higher for surgery in acute MR as there is usually recent MI.

Mitral Valve Prolapse

It is also known as Barlow's syndrome, floppy valve syndrome and midsystolic click-murmur syndrome, MVP is so-called because of displacement of one or both leaflets of MV into LA during systole. The leaflets move posteriorly and superiorly in relation to the mitral valve annulus. The causes are primary and secondary to connective tissue disorders and abnormal LV shape and size as in ASD. Secondary causes are connective tissue disorders like Marfan's syndrome (most common),

Ehlers-Danlos syndrome, pseudoxanthoma elasticum and Hurler's syndrome. In conditions like secundum atrial septal defect the left ventricular cavity size is reduced. The resulting alteration of its geometry leads to mitral valve prolapse. Mild prolapse is common and does not increase mortality. Only a thickened, elongated valve with prolapse is important as it can develop complications Table 5.1.

Symptoms and Signs

The MVP is present in 5–10 percent of population and females are affected twice as much as males. It produces atypical chest pain usually in precordial area, not related to exertional, and may be transient or prolonged and not associated with dyspnea. Other symptoms are palpitations, fatigue and dyspnea. There is no paroxysmal nocturnal dyspnea.

The patient is asthenic, with high association with scoliosis, kyphosis, and pectus excavatum and straight back syndrome. Features of Marfan's syndrome may be present. The striking feature of MVP is a click or multiple clicks and a murmur. The click is 0.14 msec after S_1 and the murmur is late systolic or in 10 percent cases pansystolic. The click may become louder and the murmur more pronounced or holosystolic on standing, after sublingual trinitroglycerine, with tachycardia or in the strain phase of the Valsalva maneuver. All these procedures lead to

Table 5.1: Complications of mitral valve prolapse (MVP)

Complication	Risk	Risk factors
Infective endocarditis	1 percent,∧ if MR	MR, thickened valve
	MR	5 percent by age 75 in males
	1 percent by age 75 in females	Male sex, obesity, hypertension, age > 50
Sudden death	MR: 0.2–1 percent	
	No MR 2/10,000	Severe MR, long QT interval, family history of MVP with complications
Embolic stroke	Rare	AF, LA enlargement, thickened valve

a decrease of left ventricular volume and cause the click to appear earlier. On the other hand, manipulations like squatting, bradycardia, administration of β-adrenergic blocking drugs and hand grip, which increase left ventricular volume, result in the click appearing later and a decrease in the systolic murmur.

Investigations

The electrocardiogram is usually normal. Nonspecific T wave and ST segment changes may be present in leads II, III and AVF and in anterolateral leads. 24 hours ambulatory ECG may reveal significant ventricular arrhythmia in a small number of patients.

Chest X-ray: Abnormalities of the bony thorax like straight back, scoliosis or kyphosis may be observed. There is no cardiac enlargement or pulmonary venous or arterial hypertension (Figs 5.7A to C).

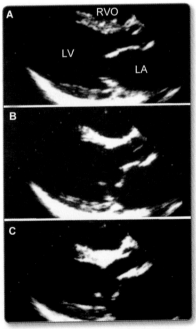

Figs 5.7A to C: MVP as seen on 2-D echocardiogram

M mode echocardiography reveals late systolic sagging of the posterior, anterior or both leaflets. In severe MVP holosystolic sagging (parachuting or hammocking) of the leaflets may be present. Two dimensional echocardiography in the apical four-chamber view gives the best delineation of the prolapsing leaflet with posterior displacement of one or both leaflets in systole below the mitral annulus. Pulsed Doppler and color flow mapping shows varying grades of mitral regurgitation.

Course and Prognosis

The disease is generally benign. Some patients may develop severe ventricular arrhythmia and sudden cardiac death. The mitral incompetence generally remains mild. However, when severe it may necessitate replacement or repair of the mitral valve. Transient ischemic episodes (due to platelet emboli) and infective endocarditis of the mitral valve may also occur. Mild MVP with normal physical findings and normal size and shale of MV is not significant.

Treatment

No treatment is generally required except prophylaxis against infective endocarditis. Beta-adrenergic blocking drugs are useful for relief of chest pain along with analgesics and reassurance.

Aortic Stenosis

The causes of aortic stenosis (AS) are rheumatic, congenital (supravalvular, valvar and subvalvar), calcified bicuspid aortic valve, degener-ative. Rheumatic AS does not occur in isolation but is present in association with aortic regurgitation or mitral valve disease. 1–2 percent of population have bicuspid aortic valve. It may become stenosed. It occurs in males and becomes symptomatic in 4–5th decade. These with tricuspid aortic valve may have a minor abnormality of the valve shape which causes turbulence and a murmur. Turbulence causes stiffening and stenosis in 5–7th decades. Those with a normal valve may also degenerate in 7–8th decade and cause AS. Vascular inflammation may also contribute to AS. The calcification is reported to be reduced by statins. Aortic sclerosis means asymptomatic AV with a murmur and reduced mobility on echocardiogram. About 5–10 percent will go on to develop stenosis in 7–8th decade.

Symptoms

AS presents as a triad of symptoms: Dyspnea, chest pain and syncope. Dyspnea is due to the low cardiac output due to the high afterload. High afterload causes hypertrophy of LV. The coronary supply is inadequate for this increased muscle mass and causes chest pain on exertion. There may be associated coronary stenosis also. The syncope or dizziness is due to low fixed output which is inadequate on exercise and cerebral perfusion reduced. It may also be due to transient tachyarrhythmia like VT or AF. LVH can cause palpitation sometimes. Later if pulmonary hypertension and RV failure occurs patient will have edema.

Signs

The blood pressure is low with reduced pulse pressure. There is a forceful and sustained apex beat which is in normal 4th intercostal space as the LVH is concentric (form outside in). A palpable thrill indicates severe stenosis. S_2 is muffled and disappears when AV is calcified. The murmur is midsystolic, diamond-shaped on phonocardiogram, like a dog's bark, short and harsh. It is well heard at the apex and the aortic area and is conducted in the neck to carotids. The murmur peaks later as the stenosis increases and late in the disease may be in whole of systole. S_3 is heard due to reduced relaxation of a hypertrophied LV (Fig. 5.8).

Investigations

ECG shows LVH with or without strain. X-ray shows a normal cardiac shadow or LVH later on. There is dilated ascending aorta, calcified valve.

Echo-Doppler study will show LVH, narrow aortic opening with doming of the valve in systole, calcification on AV if present (Fig. 5.8). The pressure gradient across the AV is the

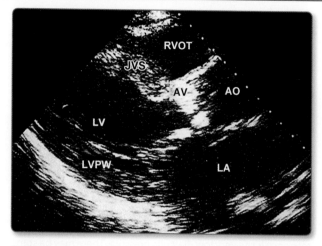

Fig. 5.8: Calcified AS on echocardiogram

main measurement and will show the severity of the stenosis. Treadmill test (TMT) is contraindicated in symptomatic AS. It may be done in asymptomatic AS and occurrence of symptoms during TMT is considered an indication for surgery. Coronary angiography is rarely done to quantify the gradient but may be required to assess coronary anatomy before surgery in patient more than 50 years of age.

Treatment

Mechanical conditions require mechanical solutions and medical therapy is no substitute for surgery. Asymptomatic patients require no therapy except endocarditis prophylaxis. Sudden cardiac death can occur in symptomatic patients. Hence surgery should be done within a month of onset of symptoms. The risk of surgery also increases with longer duration of symptoms, age of the patient, other valves or coronaries involved and other comorbid conditions like renal failure.

Surgery is the only definitive treatment. If failure develops standard antifailure treatment is started AV R is the treatment. Balloon valvotomy can be tried in very elderly or frail patients or as a bridge procedure to surgery in critically ill patients.

Aortic Regurgitation

Isolated aortic valve disease is uncommon in RHD. Chronic aortic regurgitation (AR) occurs more frequently in combination with mitral stenosis. Commissural fusion occurring as a result of rheumatic valvulitis affecting the aortic valve causes contraction of the cusps and fixes the orifice so that AR results. AR can also be because of dilated aortic root (Marfan's syndrome, ankylosing spondilitis, syphilis or ageing). AV is damaged in infective endocarditis, congenital bicuspid AV, collagen vascular disease.

Pathophysiology

Aortic regurgitation (AR) causes the ejected blood to return to the LV. This volume overload dilates LV. The large volume ejected in aorta increases the afterload and the compensatory response is the very low diastolic pressure. There may be some eccentric LVH also. Initially the dilated LV accommodates the increased blood volume and there is no increase in LVEDP. This stage may go on for years a result, the left ventricular and aortic systolic pressures rises, the aortic diastolic pressure falls very low, and the pulse pressure widens. Later on LV fails, LVEDP increases with increase in LA and pulmonary pressures.

When severe AR persists for several years myocardial hypertrophy and injury (resulting from disengagement of myocardial fibers, increased myocardial oxygen demand due to increased left ventricular mass, and reduced myocardial perfusion due to reduced aortic diastolic pressure) lead to left ventricular dysfunction. Right ventricular failure is very late and uncommon in isolated AR. Likewise, severe pulmonary arterial hypertension occurs uncommonly in this setting. In chronic severe aortic regurgitation dilatation of the mitral valve ring accompanying the left ventricular dilatation and altered geometry of the mitral valve apparatus due to altered left ventricular configuration may lead to functional mitral regurgitation, even in the absence of rheumatic mitral valvulitis. This enhances the volume overload of the left ventricle and hastens left ventricular dysfunction.

Acute AR: The cause is usually endocarditis damaging the valve cusp with sudden severe AR. Patient has pulmonary congestion with dyspnea, orthopnea. There is no time for LV to dilate and the stiff pericardium limits LV dilatation. So the pulse pressure is not wide and the blood pressure is low and murmur intensity is low.

Symptoms

Initial symptoms may be palpations due to contraction of volume overloaded LV. There may be throbbing in the neck due to large pulse pressure in carotids. Palpitations may occur due to ventricular ectopics, tachyarrhythmias late in the disease. There may be orthostatic dizziness. Patient may have angina on exertion and even at rest. Symptoms of congestive heart failure are a common late manifestation, usually occurring insidiously. Dyspnea on exertion usually remains stable for a long-time before the symptoms of more advanced left ventricular failure like paroxysmal nocturnal dyspnea develop.

Infective endocarditis may result in a rapid progress of symptoms with development of severe left ventricular failure with orthopnea and paroxysmal nocturnal dyspnea occurring in a few hours to few days, with a progressively downhill course.

Signs

AR has many signs described: The arterial pulse is characterized by a rapid rise and collapse with a markedly increased pulse pressure (Corrigan's pulse or 'water-hammer' pulse). It may have a single peak or may be bisferiens (double peak) in character. If the pulse pressure is not wide the AR is not thermodynamically significant.

The wide pulse pressure also gives rise to several characteristic peripheral signs:

1. Alternate blanching and flushing of the lightly compressed skin in the nail bed (Quincke's sign)
2. To and fro motion of the head synchronous with the cardiac cycle (de Musset's sign)
3. Dancing carotids in the neck (Corrigan's neck sign)

4. Pulsations in the uvula (Millers sign)
5. Change in size or the pupil synchronous with the cardiac cycle (Landolfi's sign).
6. Scratch on the flat surface of the skin, e.g. over the interscapular region, shows dermatographia synchronous with the cardiac cycle.
7. In severe aortic regurgitation, the diastolic pressure may be so low as to result in non disappearance of the Korotkoff sound even at zero pressure reading. In such cases, the fourth (muffling) phase of the Korotkoff sound is a reflection of the diastolic pressure.

The wide pulse pressure is also manifest as characteristic peripheral auscultatory signs:

1. Pistol-shot sounds over the femoral (Traube's sign)
2. Popliteal cuff systolic blood pressure exceeding brachial cuff systolic blood pressure by more than 20 mmHg (Hill's sign), The popliteal blood pressure usually exceeds the brachial pressure by 20–39 mmHg in mild aortic regurgitation and by 40–59 mmHg or more in severe aortic regurgitation.
3. Systolic and diastolic bruits heard over the femoral artery by lightly compressing with the edge of the stethoscope (Duroziez's sign). The characteristic diastolic component of the Duroziez's murmur is obtained by gentle distal compression.

Examination of the precordium reveals an apex bat which is displaced downward and outwards. There is parasternal heave due to hyperdynamic circulation. A systolic thrill may be palpable in suprasternal notch and along the carotids even in absence of AS due to the increased flow. The S_2 is normal or muffled especially in calcified valves. S_3 may be heard. There is a soft early diastolic murmur best heard along left sternal border in 3rd or 4th intercostal space or aortic area when there is marked aortic dilatation, it is decrescendo, better heard when patient sits stooping forward and holds his breath in expiration with the diaphragm of the stethoscope, diminished during Valsalva strain with delayed return to baseline after release (6–8 beats). The murmur is also diminished after amyl nitrate inhalation and on standing (decreased systemic vascular resistance).

A systolic ejection murmur (resembling the murmur of aortic stenosis) radiating into the carotid arteries frequently accompanies the murmur of aortic regurgitation. This results from the increased left ventricular stroke volume being ejected through the abnormal aortic valve. A systolic murmur of 'functional' mitral regurgitation also may be audible at the apex when severe regurgitation leads to marked left ventricular dilatation.

A soft, low-pitched, mid- to late-diastolic rumbling murmur, resembling the murmur of mitral stenosis, is often heard at the apex in patients with severe aortic regurgitation, even in the absence of associated mitral valve disease (Austin-Flint murmur). This murmur may be the result of (1) relative mitral stenosis resulting from the aortic regurgitant stream pushing the anterior mitral leaflet upward, (2) low-pitched vibrations of the aortic regurgitation murmur itself heard best at the apex in some patients or (3) diastolic mitral regurgitation secondary to markedly elevated left ventricular pressure. The absence of other common signs of mitral stenosis (loud S_1, opening snap, etc.) differentiate this murmur from associated mitral stenosis.

Investigations

ECG will show LVH with left axis deviation.

X-ray chest shows cardiomegaly with LV contour: Outward and downward enlargement of the left ventricle and dilatation of the ascending aorta and aortic arch. Calcification of the aortic valve is uncommon and is found only in older patients.

Echocardiogram will show enlarged LV with LVH. Aortic regurgitation produces a broad band of diastolic flutter of the anterior mitral leaflet, in the M-mode echocardiogram. The aortic root is dilated, left ventricle end-diastolic dimension is increased, and the wall motion is hyperdynamic (volume overload pattern). Increased reflectivity from the deformed aortic leaflets, leaflet fixation beginning at the bases of one or more of the aortic cusps, and multiple linear echoes along the coaptation line in diastole may be noted. Color mapping will show the regurgitant jet into LV. The severity is judged from its length. It is also useful in detecting aortic valve vegetations due to infective endocarditis. LVES size as measured by LV end systolic dimension is one of the guides to timing of surgery. When LVES dimension is 5.5 cm it is time for surgery even in absence of symptoms. Between 4–5.5 surgery is indicated if pattern is symptomatic. If LVEF falls below 55 percent or id aortic root is >55 mm surgery is advised. The rule of 55: fix AR when the LVEF falls below 55 percent, LVES diameter is > 55 mm or aortic root is > 55 mm.

Cardiac catheterization and angiography is not required unless IHD is suspected or the patient is over 50 years of age.

Medical Therapy

Vasodilator therapy is required in AR. ACE inhibiotrs, and calcium channel blocker like nifedipine has been useful. Digoxin and diuretics are given if failure symptoms are there. High systolic pressure must be treated as it favors regurgitation. Use beta-blockers with care as it may worsen HF. They cause bradycardia and prolong diastole and there is regurgitation during diastole. For same reason verapamil and diltiazem may worsen the AR. Beta-blocker is indicated in Marfan's syndrome and dilated ascending aorta to prevent dissection.

Surgery

AV replacement is the surgery of choice. In older patients bioprosthesis may be used to avoid use of anticoagulants required for mechanical valves.

Tricuspid Regurgitation

Rheumatic tricuspid regurgitation (TR) is either organic or functional secondary to pulmonary hypertension due to mitral or aortic valve disease. The later disappears on treatment with diuretics or MVR. Other causes of pulmonary hypertension like cor pulmonale and Primary pulmonary hypertension also cause TR.

Other causes are TV endocarditis especially in drug users, RV infraction, carcinoid syndrome and Ebstein's abnormality.

Pulmonary hypertension causes RV hypertrophy and dilatation resulting in TR.

Symptoms

Typically patient has anorexia, edema and abdominal distension, ascites and fatigue due to RV failure. Right hypochondrial pain may be due to hepatic engorgement and may cause jaundice.

Signs

Wasting or cardiac cachexia is particularly common in patients with tricuspid regurgitation. The jugular vein will be distended and the wave form will show prominent 'v' waves caused by RV contraction. The liver will be distended and the 'v' wave may be transmitted back causing a palpable liver. There may be pedal edema. The apical impulse is not displaced unless there is LVH. There may be a parasternal heave and a palpable pulmonary valve closure sound. The P_2 will be loud in cases of pulmonary hypertension and will be heard even on right side of sternum (Both A_2 and P_2 are heard). A RV S_3 may be heard over the sternum, well heard in inspiration. The murmur is high pitched, holosystolic and best heard along the lower left sternal border or in the xiphoid region or on right side of sternum, the intensity increases with inspiration (Carvallo's sign).

Tests

ECG shows RVH or RV overload. X-ray chest shows enlarged RA and RV. Echocardiogram shows dilated RA, RV; the TV may be deformed or dilated depending on the etiology.

Treatment

The primary cause should be treated. Isolated TR is well-tolerated for years. Diuretics may be required. If associated with mitral valve disease, it is repaired if needed at the time of mitral surgery.

Tricuspid Stenosis

Tricuspid stenosis (TS) in isolation is very rare. It is always in association with other valve involvement especially rheumatic MS.

Pathophysiology

TS causes a rise in LA pressure and a gradient across the TV. The gradient is usually much less than the one across MV in MS. The raised RA pressure is reflected in raise JVP and a prominent 'a' wave in jugular venous pulse.

Symptoms and Signs

The symptoms are also more due to the associated MS. TS itself causes low output and therefore fatigue and right-sided venous engorgement with edema, hepatic congestion and ascites.

There is a small volume pulse, low systolic and pulse pressures. S_1 is loud due to TS and associated MS. A right-sided opening snap is heard and a middiastolic rumble best heard in left lower parasternal region in 4–5th interspace, augmented by inspiration and leg elevation, the right lateral decubitus position.

Investigations

The ECG shows a prominent p wave (p pulmonale), RVH due to associated MS. AF is present in 30 percent.

The X-ray shows dilated RA; features of pulmonary arterial and venous hypertension due to associated MS. Echocardiography show a deformed TV, with reduced movements and reduced TV orifice size.

Treatment

Opening of TV with balloon or surgery are the options and the associated valvular disuse will dictate the choice of procedure.

Cardiac Arrhythmias

How is Heart Rate Controlled?

Some specialized cardiac cells situated in the sinoatrial (SA) node of the right atrium and the junctional tissue in the atrioventricular (AV) node have the property of automatic excitation. These cells act as pacemakers. The SA node has an intrinsic rhythm but is under autonomic control. Sympathetic activity accelerates it and vagal influence decreases the rate. When the rate slows down excessively, the junctional pacemaker in the AV nodal area takes over. Generally, the pacemaker in the AV node has a lower rate but in pathological states it may accelerate.

Cardiac cells possess a transmembrane action potential which consists of five phases (Fig. 6.1): phase 0; phase 1, rapid upstroke due to depolarization; phase 2, plateau; phase 3, final repolarization; phase 4, resting membrane potential and diastolic depolarization. Figure 6.1 depicts the ion fluxes associated with each phase. Each ion has its own specific channel. Ion currents pass from one cell to another without any neural input. K^+ ions determine the resting membrane potential.

Rapid influx of Na^+ ions in phase 0 is responsible for cell depolarization.

In repolarization, particularly phases 2 and 3, calcium currents play a major role.

The passage of the electrical impulse may not always be smooth. As a consequence of accessory pathways or due to block in a local area, the impulse may choose an alternate pathway. However, when the blocked zone is no longer refractory the impulse may choose to return through it, thus leading to a reentry. Reentrant mechanisms underlie most paroxysmal tachycardias. Figure 6.2 depicts the mechanism of electrical reentry when a localized area of block exists.

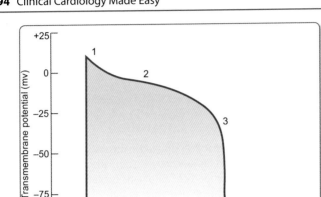

Fig. 6.1: Action potential of ventricular muscle with ionic fluxes. The four phases are depicted

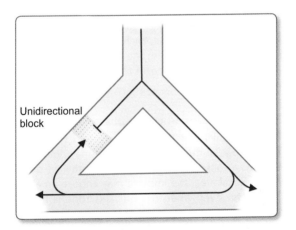

Fig. 6.2: Reentry. Unidirectional block in a branch of a Purkinje fiber alters the conduction pathway but allows reentry in the opposite direction in a slow manner (retrograde conduction)

In the clinical setting, cardiac rhythm disturbances are classified by their site of origin (Table 6.1). Identification of the P wave, its morphology and axis and its relation to the QRS complex is the first step in ECG analysis. Steep T waves may be caused by superimposition of P waves. The P-P and R-R intervals need to be measured. When the P and the QRS complexes are unrelated, the term AV dissociation is used. This may be physiological or pathological. In the latter situation, the ventricular rate is slow and the condition is commonly referred to as heart block. Failure of an expected P or QRS wave to occur may be due to a preceding impulse causing refractoriness through concealed conduction. A common example is a ventricular premature beat travelling retrogradely via the AV node in a concealed manner and delaying the subsequent atrial impulse by making the node refractory. The QRS duration may be wide during the arrhythmia; one of the causes is aberrant conduction. Finally, the QRS axis may change substantially as in ventricular tachycardia.

Disorders of Impulse Formation

Sinus Rhythm

Sinus Arrhythmia

Phasic sinus arrhythmia varying with the respiratory rate is a normal physiological phenomenon. The rate is faster at the end of inspiration, slower towards the end of expiration. The rhythm is mediated by vagal tone. It does not merit any treatment. It can be observed in young adults easily and should not be mistaken for any arrhythmia. Total absence of variations in the sinus rate is a hint of underlying heart disease; in the ICCU setting it carries an adverse prognosis.

Sinus Tachycardia

The sinus rate is generally between 100 and 140 beats/min. Physiological causes include increased sympathetic activity due to emotional excitement, exercise and pregnancy. Pathological causes include fever, thyrotoxicosis, anemia, arteriovenous fistula, congestive cardiac failure, myocardial infarction and the

Table 6.1: Classification of cardiac arrhythmias

Disorders of impulse formation

1. Sinus rhythm
   a. Sinus arrhythmia
   b. Sinus tachycardia
   c. Sinus bradycardia
   d. Sinus arrest
   e. Sinus extrasystole or bigeminy
   f. Sinus parasystole

2. Atrial rhythm
   a. Atrial escape rhythm
   b. Atrial extrasystole
   c. Atrial tachycardia
   d. Atrial flutter
   e. Atrial fibrillation
   f. Atrial parasystole

3. AV junctional (nodal) rhythm
   a. AV junctional escape rhythm
   b. AV junctional extrasystole
   c. AV junctional tachycardia
   d. AV junctional parasystole

4. Ventricular rhythm
   a. Ventricular escape-idioventricular rhythm
   b. Ventricular extrasystole
   c. Ventricular parasystole
   d. Ventricular tachycardia
   e. Ventricular flutter
   f. Ventricular fibrillation

Disorders of impulse conduction

1. SA block
   a. First degree
   b. Second degree (Wenckebach)
   c. Third degree

2. AV block
   a. First degree
   b. Second degree (Wenckebach)
   c. Third degree (complete heart block)

3. Intraventricular
   a. Right bundle branch block (RBBB)
   b. Left bundle branch block (LBBB)
   c. Fascicular blocks; left anterior, left posterior and bifascicular (trifascicular block leads to complete heart block) (LAHB, LPHB)

use of vasodilator drugs. Drugs which block the vagus nerve (e.g. atropine) and sympathomimetic drugs like adrenaline, ephedrine and isoproterenol can cause it. Excessive use of tea, coffee or tobacco may also be the underlying cause (Table 6.2).

Sinus tachycardia generally needs no treatment. Emotional factors are controlled by sedatives such as alprazolam. In some cases beta blockers may be useful. The management depends on the underlying cause.

Sinus Bradycardia

A sinus rate less than 60 beats per minute denotes sinus bradycardia. It may occur due to increased vagal tone, diminished sympathetic activity or inhibition of the S-A node. Sinus bradycardia may be physiological or pathological (Table 6.3).

Extreme bradycardia can cause dizziness, giddiness and black-outs (syncope). Asymptomatic sinus bradycardia requires no treatment. In myocardial infarction or during reperfusion following thrombolytic therapy, the slow rate may be corrected by intravenous atropine (0.3–1.2 mg). Bradycardia in symptomatic sick sinus syndrome will need the insertion of a permanent pacemaker.

Sinus Arrest

Increased vagotonia, use of vagomimetic drugs, tracheal intubation during anesthesia and tracheal aspiration may cause

Table 6.2: Important causes of sinus tachycardia

• Fever
• Anxiety
• Thyrotoxicosis
• Anemia
• Heart failure
• Pregnancy
• Pheochromocytoma
• Drugs (salbutamol, terfenadine)
• Excessive use of tea, coffee, tobacco

Table 6.3: Causes of bradycardia

1. Physiological
a. Athletes
b. Diving reflex
2. Pathological
a. Digitalis, prostigmine, etc.
b. Hypothermia
c. Obstructive jaundice
d. Myxoedema
e. Hypopituitarism
f. Beta-receptor blockade, e.g. propranolol
g. Uremia, hepatic coma
h. Increased intracranial tension
i. Hypertension
j. Myocardial infarction
k. Sick sinus syndrome

sinus arrest. In this situation long pauses are seen in the ECG due to momentary failure of the sinus node to initiate impulses. The pauses are of varying duration and not a multiple of the duration between two QRS complexes. If it causes dizziness or syncope, intravenous atropine will be beneficial.

Sinus Extrasystole
Extrasystoles arising in the SA node itself will present as premature supraventricular beats with a P wave configuration identical to the basic P wave. A similar pattern may be recognized in sinus arrhythmia; however, the pattern is related to the phases of respiration.

Sinus Parasystole
This is a rare rhythm disturbance in which an ectopic sinus node impulse is firing separately from the sinus node. The slower sinus pacemaker is protected at all times from the faster ectopic pacemaker. This dual rhythm needs no treatment.

Atrial Rhythm

Idioatrial Rhythm

When the sinus rhythm is interrupted by the failure of a sinus impulse to come through, a lower atrial pacemaker may take over. The ectopic pacemaker beats around 50/min and the P waves are inverted in leads II, III and aVf.

Atrial Extrasystole

An atrial extrasystole or premature beat arises from an ectopic atrial focus. It is premature in relation to the prevailing sinus rhythm. The ectopic beat may occur in an isolated fashion or may display a fixed relation to the sinus beat (coupled beat). A long, so called compensatory pause may exist till the next sinus beat arrives and takes over.

Atrial ectopy is due to focal irritability or a reentry. Excessive consumption of tea, coffee or tobacco can cause it. Atrial extrasystoles are seen in organic heart disease, thyrotoxicosis, atrial septal defect (ASD), chronic lung disease and postoperatively. Ectopy is recognized by the premature and abnormal shape of the P wave preceding the early QRS complex. The compensatory pause is incomplete, i.e. the interval between the sinus P wave before the premature beat and the P wave of the sinus beat following it is less than twice the prevailing cycle length of the normal sinus rhythm. Atrial extrasystoles may be numerous and in some cases multifocal. Such a situation heralds sustained atrial tachycardia. The management is directed to the underlying condition.

Atrial or Supraventricular Tachycardia

A rapid succession of six or more consecutive ectopic atrial beats constitutes an atrial or supraventricular tachycardia (SVT). If it is of sudden origin and transient in nature, the SVT is termed as paroxysmal. Repeated episodes of SVT may be seen in cases where there is an accessory pathway like the bundle of Kent in the Wolff-Parkinson-White (WPW) syndrome (Fig. 6.3).

Increased automaticity of the atrial pacemaker due to excess of tea, coffee, alcohol and tobacco can result in SVT. Thyrotoxicosis must be kept in mind. ASD, rheumatic

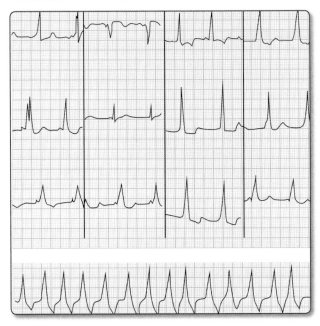

Fig. 6.3: Wolft-Parkinson-White syndrome

heart disease (RHD), ischemic heart disease (IHD) and cardiomyopathy may present with SVT. Anxiety, sweating, pounding of the chest, abdominal distension and nausea may result. Following termination of the attack there may be polyuria. Syncope, cerebral hypoxia and, rarely, death may result. The heart rate is 140–220/min, and may be abruptly reduced by vagal stimulation, Valsalva maneuver or immersion of the face in ice-cold water (diving reflex).

In the presence of digitalis toxicity (Table 6.4) the SVT may present with a 2:1 ventricular response [paroxysmal atrial tachycardia (PAT) with block]. This may mimic atrial flutter, but in flutter the baseline is constantly undulating and has a saw-tooth appearance; also, the atrial rate in flutter is above 250/min.

Table 6.4: Digitalis toxicity

Cardiac
1. Sinus bradycardia
2. Ventricular premature beats
3. Bigeminy
4. Paroxysmal atrial tachycardia (PAT)
5. Ventricular tachycardia
6. Ventricular fibrillation
Extracardiac
1. Nausea, vomiting
2 Diarrhea
3. Gynecomastia
Management
1. Stop digoxin and measure electrolytes, blood urea, serum creatinine and digoxin levels
2. Correct potassium and dehydration
3. Give IV atropine injections (0.6 mg) or do temporary pacing if severe bradycardia
4. For PAT, use beta-blockers and for ventricular tachycardia, use lignocaine
5. For ventricular fibrillation, use DC defibrillator

Vagal stimulation by means of carotid sinus massage or by Valsalva maneuver is the first step in the management. If there is no response, the drugs of choice are adenosine and verapamil given intravenously (5–10 mg). Digitalis given intravenously is a good alternative when verapamil and DC countershock have failed. Propranolol, 0.1 mg/kg given intravenously, may be useful. Flecainide and encainide are very useful when myocardial contractility is not compromised. Amiodarone, 5 mg/kg as an IV infusion, given over 20 minutes to 2 hours is effective. Diltiazem may be given as a bolus, 25 mg IV, followed by a drip containing 125 mg in 100 mL of dextrose-saline.

Rapid atrial pacing is a useful alternative. Currently, electro-ablation of the abnormal pathway or focus is the method of choice. In PAT with block, digitalis is stopped and potassium chloride IV is given. Diphenylhydantoin counteracts digitalis toxicity.

Atrial Flutter

The atrial rate is 220–350 beats/min. The ventricles respond to every second, third or fourth atrial beat due to physiological AV block. The etiology is the same as in PAT.

During vagal stimulation or administration of digitalis, the flutter rate may change from 2 : 1 to 3 : 1 or 4 : 1.

Synchronized DC shock is the treatment of choice. A low energy level of 100–200 Joules may be all that is necessary. Intravenous digoxin is beneficial. Quinidine may be tried but not without prior digitalization; otherwise, flutter with a dangerous 1:1 conduction may occur. Acute episodes of flutter may respond to IV propranolol or verapamil. It is a good policy to give anticoagulant prior to DC conversion when the atrial flutter occurs in mitral stenosis, to avoid the risk of embolism from a clot in the left atrium.

Atrial Fibrillation (AF)

The heart beats are irregularly irregular and there is a total lack of coordinated and sequential activation of the atria. Many of the rapid atrial impulses are blocked by the AV node. Some impulses however pass through and activate the ventricles. Concealed conduction may occur in addition.

Atrial fibrillation may be paroxysmal or persistent. In lone atrial fibrillation, no organic cause can be detected. Atrial fibrillation can be part of the "tachy-brady" syndrome in sick sinus disease. Longstanding AF is seen in RHD, especially mitral stenosis, ischemic heart disease, thyrotoxicosis, cardiomyopathy, chronic obstructive lung disease, ASD and postoperatively (Table 6.5).

The rapid ventricular response may be blocked by digitalis. Verapamil and diltiazem are useful in increasing the AV block and 'regularizing' the response. DC countershock may be

Table 6.5: Important causes of atrial fibrillation

1. Rheumatic heart disease (mitral stenosis)
2. Ischemic heart disease
3. Hyperthyroidism
4. Sinoatrial disease
5. Hypertension
6. Pericarditis
7. Lone atrial fibrillation (idiopathic)
8. Cardiomyopathy, myocarditis
9. Alcohol
10. Congenital heart disease (ASD)

tried but the results are transient. Normal sinus rhythm may be restored with quinidine, 200–600 mg 2 hourly for 5 doses, with a maintenance dose of 200 mg three to four times a day. Procainamide is an alternative; frequently, large doses may be necessary. Propranolol and verapamil are useful in controlling the ventricular rate. In difficult cases amiodarone may be tried. Long-term anticoagulation should be considered so as to prevent thromboembolic complications. Prior to elective conversion of AF, the patient should be on anticoagulants.

Atrial Parasystole
A parasystolic focus can originate anywhere in the atrium. The fixed pattern of firing identities it. No specific treatment is needed.

AV Junctional Rhythm
Idionodal Rhythm
Idionodal or junctional rhythm is a 'nodal escape' rhythm when the sinus impulse fails to arrive at the appointed time. The ventricular rate is 40–60/min. The clue is in the P wave morphology; it is inverted in leads II, III and aVf. It may be lost in the QRS complex or follow the QRS complex when there is retrograde conduction.

AV junctional rhythm may be due to digitalis toxicity. It is also seen in inferior wall infarction. Latent sinus node dysfunction may present as an AV junctional rhythm first. Later, various disturbances of sinus rhythm may show up if the junctional rate is less than 50/min; atropine 0.3–1.2 mg IV or isoproterenol may be given.

AV Junctional Extrasystoles

These arise in an ectopic AV junctional focus and are premature in time. The P wave is inverted in leads II, III and aVf, and the P-R duration is less than 0.12 sec. No treatment is necessary.

AV Junctional Tachycardia

In the paroxysmal form, the ventricular rate is between 140 and 200/min. This is also called extrasystolic junctional tachycardia. The nonparoxysmal form is at a slower rate of 100–140/min. Usually this is due to digitalis toxicity. It may be seen in acute rheumatic fever and myocardial infarction.

AV Junctional Parasystole

An ectopic beat of junctional origin independent of the basic rhythm, with mathematically related interectopic intervals, is a clue to this condition. It is rare and needs no treatment.

Ventricular Rhythm

Ventricular Escape Rhythm

This is due to failure of the sinus impulse to reach and extinguish the site of the ectopic ventricular pacemaker. This can happen, for example, in sinus bradycardia. The escape beat has no preceding P wave and the QRS complex is slurred.

Accelerated idioventricular rhythm is particularly seen after coronary reperfusion with thrombolytic therapy. No specific treatment is needed.

Ventricular Extrasystole

It arises in an ectopic ventricular focus and is premature in time. Ventricular extrasystoles may occur in healthy individuals. In young women it may be due to mitral valve prolapse.

Ventricular extrasystoles can be seen in all forms of organic heart disease. Drugs, alcohol, and overuse of tea, coffee or tobacco may precipitate these premature beats.

Ventricular extrasystoles are followed by a compensatory pause. They can occur in early or late diastole. Occasionally they may be interpolated between two normal QRS complexes without a compensatory pause. A ventricular extrasystole can occur with a fixed coupling to the previous QRS complex.

A ventricular extrasystole invariably travels retrograde through the AV node and cause refractoriness due to concealed conduction. This is why the next sinus impulse is unable to traverse the AV node. A compensatory pause must necessarily follow.

Benign ventricular extrasystoles usually disappear on exercise. Multiform, bigeminal, exercise-induced extrasystoles indicate organic heart disease. Salvos of extrasystoles usually presage ventricular tachycardia.

Benign ventricular extrasystoles are best left alone. Correction of electrolyte imbalance, withdrawal of digitalis if there is toxicity, and removal of stimulants like tea, coffee and tobacco are helpful measures. The usual therapy of pathologically significant extrasystoles consists of quinidine, procainamide, diisopyramide or mexeiletine. For resistant ventricular extrasystoles, amiodarone is the drug of choice. When they occur in salvos, intravenous lidocaine 1 mg/kg IV is the drug of choice. Other useful drugs are verapamil and diphenylhydantoin; the former is particularly effective in ventricular tachycardia which presents as right bundle branch block (RBBB) with left axis deviation and the latter is recommended in the presence of digitalis toxicity.

Ventricular Parasystole

An ectopic ventricular focus may fire in a mathematically precise manner without any interference from the prevailing rhythm. Unidirectional entry block protects the parasystolic focus. Rarely, a succession of parasystoles may present as a tachycardia. The prognosis of ventricular parasystolic tachycardia is benign in comparison to ventricular tachycardia.

Ventricular Tachycardia

A rapid succession of three or more consecutive beats constitutes ventricular tachycardia. The rate is over 100/min. Focal repetitive discharges or reentry is the mechanisms for its origin. Ischemic heart disease, myocarditis, cardiomyopathies, RHD and mitral valve prolapse are the usual causes. Drugs can be proarrhythmic and precipitate ventricular tachycardia (Figs 6.4 and 6.5).

A sudden rise in ventricular rate with bizarre QRS complexes, hypotension and intermittent cannon 'a' waves in the neck with varying intensity of heart sounds, suggests the diagnosis.

Serial ECG tracings will reveal the same form of the ectopic ventricular complex in the tachycardia. There is AV dissociation with occasional fusion beats. Capture beats may also be noted when sinus beats with critical timing 'capture' the ventricles. The following morphologies of the QRS pattern suggest a ventricular origin, in contrast to supraventricular origin with

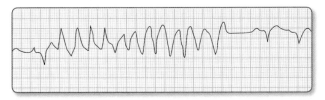

Fig. 6.4: ECG showing paroxysmal ventricular tachycardia

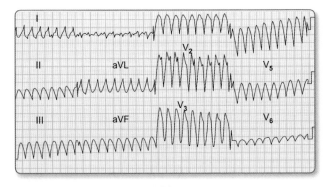

Fig. 6.5: ECG showing ventricular tachycardia

aberration: (1) left bundle branch block (LBBB) pattern, (2) RBBB with initial R taller than R′, (3) concordant QRS pattern across V_1 to V_6, (4) QS pattern in V_1 to V_6 and (5) QRS duration greater than 0.14 sec.

Synchronized DC countershock is the treatment of choice. Following this, IV lidocaine is started at a dose of 1–3 mg/min. If countershock facilities are not immediately available lidocaine may be given in bolus doses of 50–75 mg and followed by an IV drip. Procainamide is given as 50 mg/min until a total of 2 g is reached. Propranolol may be given slowly IV in doses of 1 mg every 2 minutes. Other drugs include IV diisopyramide and mexeletine. In difficult cases, IV amiodarone 300 mg has proved to be useful. Bretylium tosylate, 5–10 mg/kg as a loading dose followed by an IV infusion at a rate of 0.5–4.0 mg/min, is also a valuable alternative.

Surgical interruption or transcatheter ablation of the re-entry pathway and aneurysmectomy are sometimes needed to treat refractory cases. If the QRS complexes have a varying shape, the ventricular tachycardia is known as pleomorphic. An important variant is torsade de pointes where the QRS complexes have a twisting nature with a cyclical variation in axis; this is always associated with prolonged QT interval. This variety of ventricular tachycardia responds best to IV isoproterenol and electrolyte correction.

Ventricular Flutter

The ECG looks like a sine wave. The ventricular activation is very rapid. It may degenerate into ventricular fibrillation and needs urgent therapy along the lines of ventricular tachycardia.

Ventricular Fibrillation

Chaotic incoordinated ventricular depolarization characterizes ventricular fibrillation. It is seen in severe organic heart disease, myocardial infarction, hereditary QT prolongation syndromes, hypothermia, hyperkalemia, mitral valve prolapse, general anesthesia and in electrocution (Fig. 6.6).

This is one of the forms of cardiac arrest. Electrical defibrillation is the treatment of choice. Resuscitative measures

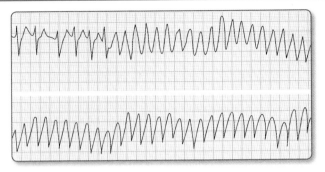

Fig. 6.6: Ventricular fibrillation

involving rhythmic manual compression of the chest, mouth-to-mouth respiration and proper maintenance of the airway are mandatory.

Treatment
Antiarrhythmic Drugs
Antiarrhythmic drugs can be classified electrophysiologically into those that block sodium, potassium or calcium channels and those that block adrenergic beta-receptors. The generally accepted classification is by Vaughan Williams (Table 6.6).

Antiarrhythmic drugs should be used judiciously with frequent monitoring of ECG and serum potassium and magnesium concentration. They can be proarrhythmic under certain circumstances. This is particularly true with Class I anti-arrhythmic agents.

Ablation Therapy
Electrical ablation of the His bundle using a platinum-tipped catheter is carried out for refractory supraventricular tachycardia with a rapid ventricular response. It can also be used in WPW syndrome to interrupt the accessory pathway, especially a right posteroseptal pathway near the coronary ostium. Laser ablation of ventricular foci for tachycardia has recently been introduced. Selective embolization of the AV

Table 6.6: Classification of antiarrhythmic drugs

Drugs	Dosage
Class 1 A	
Quinidine	600–1600 mg/day in 2–4 divided doses
Procainamide	750–6000 mg/day in 3–4 divided doses; IV 5–15 mg/kg loading over 20–60 min, 5 mg/min as maintenance
Disopyramide	200–800 mg/day in 2 or 3 divided doses
Ethmozine	600–900 mg/day in 3 or 4 divided doses
Class I B	
Lidocaine	IV 1–3 mg/kg loading over 20 min and 1–4 mg/min as maintenance
Mexeletine	600–1000 mg/day in 3–4 divided doses
Phenytoin	14 mg/kg loading, 200–400 mg/day in 1–2 divided doses; IV 50–100 mg every 5 min to a maximum of 1000 mg
Tocainide	80–1800 mg/day in 2–4 divided doses
Class I C	
Encainide	75–200 mg/day in 3–4 divided doses
Flecainide	100–200 mg twice daily; IV 1–2 mg/kg over 10–20 minutes
Class II	
Propranolol	40–240 mg/day in divided doses; IV 0.5 to 1.0 mg every 5 minutes to a maximum of 0.2 mg/kg
Acebutolol	400–1200 mg/day in 2 divided doses
Esmolol	500 µg/kg/min bolus followed by 5–6 mg/min infusion
Class III	
Amiodarone	800–1600 mg/day in 4 divided doses, then 100–400 mg/day as maintenance IV 50–100 mg/kg in 20 min to 2 hours
Bretylium	IV 5–10 mg/kg loading, 5 mg/kg every 6 hours or 0.5 to 4.0 mg/min as continuous infusion
Sotalol	120–240 mg/day in divided doses
Class IV	
Verapamil	160–480 mg/day in four divided doses; IV 3–10 mg bolus over 2–3 min, repeated in 30 min; 0.125 mg/min as maintenance infusion
Diltiazem	90–180 mg/day in three divided doses
Other	
Digoxin	0.125–0.375 mg/day; IV 0.25–0.5 mg initially followed by 0.1–0.3 mg every 4–8 h to a maximum of 1 mg in 24 h
Adenosine	IV bolus 6 mg with saline flush, repeat 9–12 mg minutes later

nodal artery has also been successively carried out. Recently, radiofrequency-induced discharge has been found to be most effective in ablating the AV node.

Surgically the endocardial tissue may be excised, isolated or interrupted by an encircling incision. This has been done for refractory ventricular tachycardias.

Disorders of Impulse Conduction

Impulses generated from the pacemaker cells in the SA node spread out through the atrium and are transmitted to the AV node. From here the impulse travels via the His bundle to the Purkinje system of conduction tissue in the ventricles. The conducting fibers in the ventricles can be grouped into anterior and posterior fascicles. Transmission of an impulse may be blocked at any level, resulting in atrioventricular or intraventricular conduction defects.

Heart Block
Sinoatrial Block

SA block can exist as first degree, second degree or third degree block. The SA node fails to discharge intermittently. Each time this happens, a complete cardiac cycle is missed. Both atrial and ventricular complexes are missing. SA block is often present in the 'sick sinus syndrome'. Normally, SA block needs no treatment. Pacemaker therapy is indicated if it occurs as part of the sick sinus syndrome.

Atrioventricular Block

In first degree AV block, the P-R interval is prolonged beyond 0.20 sec. Apart from rheumatic fever, ischemic heart disease and cardiomyopathy, drugs like digitalis, verapamil and beta-blockers can cause P-R prolongation because of the AV delay, the first heart sound is soft and the jugular venous pulse exhibits a prolonged a-c interval.

In second degree heart block or partial heart block, some of the atrial impulses fail to get past to the ventricles. This leads to dropped beats.

In Mobitz type I block, there is progressive lengthening of successive P-R intervals till a beat is dropped (Wenckebach cycle).

In Mobitz type II block, the P-R interval is constant but intermittently some P waves are not conducted. The pathology is situated in the infra-Hisian region and it is a more serious condition than Mobitz block (Fig. 6.7).

Second degree heart block is recognized by a slow pulse which may change suddenly as the degree of heart block alters. The ECG will reveal an A-V block generally in the ratio of 1:1 or 3:1.

Complete Heart Block

Complete heart block (CHB) has a pathological origin (Table 6.7).

In CHB, there is total dissociation of the atrial and ventricular complexes. In an earlier stage (advanced heart block) some atrial beats may capture the ventricles (Fig. 6.7).

In congenital heart block, the QRS complexes are not wide and the heart rate is around 60/min (a slow rate in the pediatric

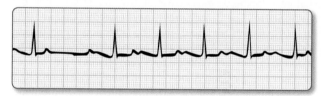

Fig. 6.7: Mobitz I block

Table 6.7: Important causes of complete heart block

I. Congenital
II. Acquired
a. Fibrosis of the septal summit (Lev's disease)
b. Myocardial infarction
c. Inflammatory condition like aortic root abscess, Chagas' disease, sarcoidosis, tuberculosis
d. Trauma
e. Drug induced, e.g. digoxin

age group). In CHB of the acquired type, the block is at the infra-Hisian level. It may be trifascicular in origin.

Venous cannon waves occur in the neck whenever the atrium contracts simultaneously with the ventricle. The closed tricuspid valve reflects the 'a' wave into the neck. Loud cannon sounds (S_1) are intermittently heard when the P-R distance is short. Cannon waves and cannon sounds do not occur at the same time.

Episodes of ventricular asystole can cause cardiac syncope (Adams-Stokes attacks). Long arrests can cause convulsions, cerebral anoxia and even death. Sudden recovery with re-appearance of the heart beat is characteristic. This does not occur in epilepsy.

Treatment

First degree heart block is managed by removing any offending drugs and treating the cause.

Second degree heart block of Mobitz type II is sinister in nature. Atropine, 0.6 mg IV, is useful. An IV drip of isoprenaline, 2 mg in 500 mL 5 percent dextrose, may be needed. Orciprenaline and hydralazine are also useful. The latter acts by producing reflex tachycardia. A temporary pacing electrode should be inserted in the right ventricle by a transvenous route.

Permanent pacing is indicated in long-standing Mobitz II and in complete AV block, even if the patient is asymptomatic; the only exception is in congenital CHB when the heart rate exceeds 50/min. Pacemaker therapy is used with restraint, the chief indication being the occurrence of symptoms.

Intraventricular conduction defects will result in RBBB, LBBB, LAHB, and LPHB (Table 6.8).

Pacemakers

The artificial cardiac pacemaker is an electronic device used to deliver repetitive electrical stimuli to the heart in order to treat bradycardias as well as tachycardias (Fig. 6.8).

The pacing lead is a steerable insulated wire and is introduced via the cephalic, subclavian or external jugular vein during cardiac catheterization. It may be also placed via the femoral

Table 6.8: Important causes of bundle branch block

Right bundle branch block	Left bundle branch block
• May be normal	• Ischemic heart disease (IHD)
• Atrial septal defect (incomplete RBBB)	• Aortic valve disease
• R ventricular overload	• Hypertension
• IHD	• Cardiomyopathy
• Myocarditis	• Myocarditis

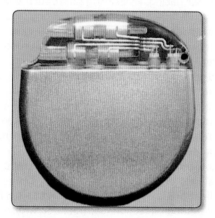

Fig. 6.8: The pacemaker

vein. Rarely, the lead may be placed in the esophagus. Modern pulse generators are compact and multi-programmable. The modes of pacing are designated by a five-letter notation. For pacing and sensing the terminology is: V = ventricle, A = atrium, D = double chamber, O = none. For the mode of response: I = inhibited, T = triggered, D = double, R = rate responsive and O = none. Modern developments include built-in defibrillatory activity for ventricular tachycardia.

Temporary pacing is indicated in conditions in which symptomatic bradycardia is present or likely to occur. These include the following situations:

a. During right heart catheterization with preexisting left bundle branch block
b. During percutaneous transluminal coronary angioplasty
c. Administration of drugs causing bradycardia
d. Bradycardia following thrombolytic therapy
e. Prior to implantation of a permanent pacemaker
f. Bradycardia with heart failure.

In the setting of acute myocardial infarction AV temporary pacing may be needed when various conduction disturbances occur. Type II AV block, advanced AV block and CHB are indications for pacing. Preexisting bifascicular block in the setting of acute anterior infarction is a strong indication for prophylactic pacing.

Permanent pacing is indicated in the following conditions:

a. Complete heart attack
b. Second degree AV block following infarction
c. Chronic bi- or trifascicular block with symptomatic bradycardia
d. Sinus node dysfunction (sick sinus) with bradycardia
e. Hypertensive carotid sinus syndrome with recurrent syncopal attacks or asystole
f. Symptomatic ventricular tachycardia not responding to medical treatment.

Complications of pacing include cardiac perforation, arrhythmias, emboli, infection, lead fracture and displacement of the pulse generator.

Pacemakers can be inhibited by electromagnetic fields involving diathermy, cautery, transformers, magnetic detectors, mobile, telephone and motors.

The pacemaker syndrome is manifested by light-headedness, syncope or episodic weakness due to long cycles of AV asynchrony during ventricular (VVI) pacing. It can also occur with rate-responsive pacemakers if the setting for the threshold is inappropriate. For these reasons and the risk of atrial fibrillation with its attendant problems, DDDR pacing (dual chamber, rate responsive) is the preferred method. Such pacemakers are versatile, allowing different programs which can make pacing as physiological as possible.

Pacemakers may also be used for terminating supraventricular or ventricular tachycardias. Generally these methods involve underdrive or overdrive pacing. Paired or coupled pacing is also employed. The main object is to produce refractoriness in the pathway of the arrhythmia.

Recent developments include rate-responsive pacing in which physiological stimuli such as changes in blood pH, oxygen saturation, muscular activity, Q-T interval, etc. are used to program the heart rate according to physical activity.

The automatic implantable cardioverter defibrillator (AICD) is a specially designed unit which senses ventricular tachycardia and provides defibrillation. It is highly effective in the management of drug-resistant and malignant ventricular arrhythmias.

Myocardial diseases or cardiomyopathies can be due to increase in myocardial fibers (hypertrophy) or their stretching (dilated) or failure to relax (restrictive) in absence of other known cardiovascular abnormality like hypertension, IHD, valvular, congenital or pericardial heart diseases.

The WHO has classified cardiomyopathies into three subtypes according to anatomic and pathophysiologic features (Fig. 7.1).

a. Dilated/congestive cardiomyopathy
b. Hypertrophic cardiomyopathy
c. Restrictive cardiomyopathy.

Hypertrophic Cardiomyopathy

Hypertrophic cardiomyopathy (HCM) is a syndrome with LVH without pressure overload as the common pathophysiology. About 60 percent are inherited and the remainder sporadic. Several genetic defects may contribute in familial variety the commonest is idiopathic hypertrophic subaortic stenosis (IHSS) also called hypertrophic obstructive cardiomyopathy (HOCM). There is septal hypertrophy with disorientation and histologically abnormal fibers. The symptoms are due to four causes: Diastolic dysfunction, aortic outflow tract obstruction, myocardial ischemia and arrhythmias.

Pathophysiology and Findings

The obstruction is below the aortic valve which itself is normal causing a pressure gradient below the aortic valve. The hypertrophied septum crowds the LV outflow tract. The high velocity blood flow across the narrowed outflow causes a venturi effect pulling the AML towards the septum, the so-called systolic anterior motion (SAM) of MV that is one of the

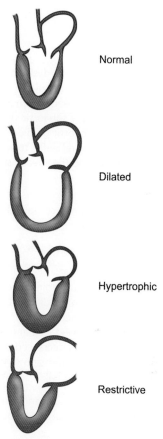

Normal

Dilated

Hypertrophic

Restrictive

Fig. 7.1: Types of cardiomyopathy

hallmarks of IHSS (best seen on echocardiography). The SAM causes the pressure gradient. In some there is no SAM and no pressure gradient and these are also called asymmetrical septal hypertrophy (ASH) rather than IHSS.

Diastolic Dysfunction

Most patients have diastolic ventricular dysfunction, and in fact it is the chief abnormality in these patients. Diastolic dysfunction is due to both impaired relaxation and chamber stiffness.

Systolic Dysfunction

Initially it was thought that systolic dysfunction, because of dynamic obstruction to the left ventricular outflow, is the chief abnormality in HCM. It has now been shown that a majority of patients in fact do not have any subaortic gradient either at rest or on provocation. The subaortic gradient occurs because of movement of the anterior mitral leaflet towards the septum in systole, which further narrows the already small outflow.

Symptoms

The presentation of HCM varies from completely asymptomatic to complete disablement.

Dyspnea occurs because of raised left ventricular filling pressures.

Chest pain is usually like atypical angina (occurs at rest, prolonged, not relieved by nitrates, more diffuse) but the predominant mechanism is myocardial ischemia. Myocardial ischemia occurs both because of increased demand and decreased supply. Coronary blood supply is decreased because of small coronary vessel disease and compression of intramyocardial vessels (especially septal perforators).

Palpitation because of supraventricular and ventricular rhythm disturbances is quite common. Atrial fibrillation occurs in 5–10 percent of patients.

Syncope can occur either because of hemodynamic factors or because of rhythm disturbances.

Sudden death: The annual mortality rate is about 2–3 percent. Although some patients die of chronic progressive congestive heart failure or peripheral embolism, most patients die suddenly due to arrhythmias like supraventricular and ventricular tachyarrhythmias, bradyarrhythmia, aberrant atrioventricular conduction and complete heart block.

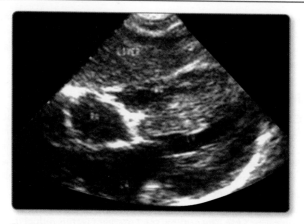

Fig. 7.2: Echocardiogram in hypertrophic cardiomyopathy showing septal hypertrophy

Signs

The murmur and the gradient are increased with lower LV volume. So maneuvers which cause reduced LV volume like standing after squatting, the strain phase of Valsalva maneuver, and amylnitrate will accentuate the murmur and SAM.

Unlike in valvular AS, the classical finding of HCM is a late systolic murmur best audible along the left lower sternal edge or between the left sternal edge and the apex. The systolic murmur is not radiated to neck and is caused by MR and turbulence in LVOT. The initial upstroke in IHHS is brisk as the obstruction is midsystolic when LV volume is reduced whereas in valvular AS the initial upstroke is delayed. Carotid artery palpation reveals a brisk upstroke and usually a notch in the upstroke (bisferiens). In both due to stiff LV there is S_4 gallop and an apical a wave.

Cardiac size is usually normal on chest X-ray. There is left atrial enlargement and features of pulmonary venous congestion.

ECG abnormalities are nonspecific ST and T wave changes, left ventricular hypertrophy, left axis deviation, prominent and deep Q waves reflecting abnormal septal depolarization in the inferior and lateral precordial leads, short PR interval and very rarely Wolff-Parkinson-White syndrome and left atrial enlargement (Table 7.1).

Management

Competitive exercise should be stopped. Hypovolemia and hypotension should be avoided. Inotropic agents like digoxin, excessive diuretics and vasodilators should not be used. None of the treatments have shown to improve survival though some relive symptoms. Drugs that block contractility (verapamil, beta-blockers, and disopyramide) cause ventricular dilatation widening outflow tract and reducing outflow velocity which minimizes SAM. The outflow tract gradient is thus reduced.

Beta-blockers are the most extensively used drugs in HCM. They act by their negative inotropic action and by decreasing exercise-induced tachycardias. They are effective in providing symptomatic relief in most patients. They have no effect on long-term prognosis and do not prevent sudden cardiac death. Similarly they have not been shown to improve diastolic dysfunction.

Table 7.1: Echo in hypertrophic cardiomyopathy

i. Left ventricular hypertrophy, septal hypertrophy and asymmetrical septal hypertrophy (Fig. 7.2).
ii. Systolic anterior motion of anterior and/or posterior mitral leaflets.
iii. Small left ventricular cavity with hyperdynamic systolic function and apical cavity obliteration during systole.
iv. Decreased septal motion with reduced systolic thickening of the interventricular septum (IVS) with generally normal or increased motion of the left ventricular posterior wall (LVPW).
v. Partial closure of the aortic valve in midsystole in those patients who have systolic gradients.
vi. Left atrial enlargement.

Calcium-channel blockers like verapamil, nifedipine and diltiazem have been used in patients who are nonresponsive to adequate doses of beta blockers. Rarely, verapamil may cause pulmonary edema or sudden death in patients with HCM.

Disopyramide, a class IA antiarrhythmic drug, acts predominantly by its negative inotropic effect. It can be combined with calcium-channel blockers but has not been shown to prevent sudden death or alter long-term prognosis.

Amiodarone is the drug of choice for symptomatic and asymptomatic supraventricular and ventricular arrhythmias.

Diuretics should be used cautiously for control of pulmonary venous congestion; excessive diuresis should be avoided.

Digoxin is used only for control of ventricular rate in atrial fibrillation. It can be used safely during the dilated stage of HCM.

Catheter ablation of septal muscle with local infusion of alcohol a septal perforating artery has shown good results with the only complication of heart block. This might replace surgical procedure.

Surgery
Two surgical methods have been used in patients with HCM:
a. *Septal myotome/myectomy*: This acts by broadening the left ventricular outflow tract. It is associated with a mortality of 5–10 percent and hence is presently not offered to asymptomatic or minimally symptomatic patients
b. *Mitral valve replacement*: The mitral valve is replaced by prosthetic valve in patients who have severe mitral regurgitation.

Genetic Counseling
As a majority of cases (55%) are familial, genetic counseling is important.

Complications
Atrial fibrillation
It is a medical emergency as it can precipitate pulmonary edema, congestive heart failure or both. Immediate cardioversion is

usually required. Recently amiodarone has been found to be useful in conversion of atrial fibrillation (AF) and maintenance of sinus rhythm.

Myocardial Ischemia
Infective endocarditis (IE)
The risk of IE is 5–10 percent. Infective endocarditis (IE) usually occurs on the mitral valve, on contact lesions of the interventricular septum or on the aortic valve. Hence all patients with HCM should receive IE prophylaxis.

Congestive cardiac failure
Around 5 percent of patients with HCM undergo progressive ventricular dilatation and congestive cardiac failure. This is usually preterminal.

Prognosis: Annual mortality is low at about 2–3 percent. Half die as sudden cardiac death (SCD). SCD can be the presenting feature, so all family members should be screened with echocardiography.

Dilated Cardiomyopathy

Dilated cardiomyopathy (DCM) is characterized by dilatation of cardiac chambers and systolic dysfunction manifesting clinically as congestive cardiac failure. A variety of etiological factors have been implicated in the causation of DCM. However, in the majority of cases, no identifiable cause can be found.

Idiopathic DCM is a progressive disease with around 75 percent of patients succumbing within 5 years after diagnosis. Occasionally, deterioration is much slower with prolonged survival. A few instances are reported when distinctive clinical improvement occurred and the cardiac size regressed. DCM has been seen in all age groups. Children have a particularly grave prognosis, though a minority may show some improvement.

Etiology
The syndrome of DCM may occur because of a number of infectious, toxic and metabolic factors. It is thought that some

patients who suffer from viral myocarditis may progress to DCM, a contention not convincing in a majority of cases. Viral infection theoretically can cause myocardial dysfunction either by inciting an inflammatory reaction or by triggering an autoimmune response. Occasionally, DCM occurs in families (familial DCM).

Clinical Manifestations
History
Patients may be asymptomatic for year despite having dilated ventricles. In some, precipitating factors like viral infection bring it to notice. DCM is seen at all ages though the commonest age of presentation is 20–40 years.

Breathlessness, the predominant symptom, initially occurs only on exertion but later progresses to orthopnea and paroxysmal nocturnal dyspnea. Fatigue and weakness are also common and reflect decreased cardiac output. Symptoms of congestive heart failure like swelling of feet and abdomen and right upper quadrant pain (because of congestive hepato-megaly) are late symptoms.

Chest pain occurs in some patients and is usually atypical. Typical anginal chest pain suggests coexisting coronary artery disease.

Palpitation because of supraventricular and ventricular arrhythmia is occasionally the presenting symptom. These patients also have a very high incidence of thromboembolism in both the systemic and pulmonary circulations. Sometimes a routine chest X-ray showing cardiac enlargement may bring the disease to notice.

Physical Examination
This usually reveals variable degree of cardiac enlargement and congestive heart failure. Systolic BP is usually normal or low, with narrow pulse pressure. There may be pulsus alternans in later stages, reflecting severe left ventricular dysfunction. Jugular venous pressure is elevated, with prominent 'v' waves and 'y' collapse when tricuspid regurgitation is present. There may be hepatomegaly with systolic pulsations in the liver, edema of feet and ascites.

Protodiastolic gallop (S_3) may be palpable at the apex. In an occasional patient features of moderate to severe pulmonary hypertension are seen. S_3 and S_4 are commonly audible, and summation gallop may be heard during tachycardia. Murmurs of mitral or tricuspid regurgitations are audible quite commonly. Mitral regurgitation occurs because of altered geometry of the left ventricle which causes malalignment of papillary muscles. On the other hand, tricuspid regurgitation occurs because of tricuspid annular dilatation.

Investigations

Chest X-ray usually shows cardiomegaly; features of pulmonary venous congestion because of left ventricular failure may be seen. Small pleural effusion may be seen. The superior vena cava and azygous vein are dilated once congestive heart failure supervenes. One should also look for evidence of pulmonary infarction. Calcification of valvular or vascular structures is extremely uncommon and its presence should arouse suspicion of another disease.

ECG commonly shows sinus tachycardia. Almost all types of supraventricular and ventricular tachyarrhythmias and conduction disturbances have been described. ST-T changes are quite common. LBBB is the commonest conduction abnormality.

Echocardiography is useful for quantifying left ventricular dysfunction and excluding pericardial, valvular and ischemic heart disease. Echocardiography usually reveals global left ventricular hypokinesia, large ventricular cavity and increased E point septal separation. Both atria are dilated and in later stages RV is also dilated (Fig. 7.3).

Small pericardial effusion may be seen. Doppler confirms and quantifies the presence of atrioventricular regurgitation. Thrombi in various chambers of the heart are also commonly detected in DCM.

Cardiac catheterization and coronary angiography may be required in a few patients to exclude coronary artery disease as a cause of cardiac failure.

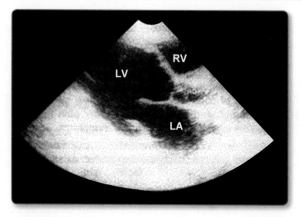

Fig. 7.3: Typical 2D echo of dilated cardiomyopathy showing dilated LV and large LA

Management

The management of DCM predominantly involves management of heart failure (For details, refer chapter on congestive heart failure).

Exercise

Traditional advice has been to avoid exercise and maintain a sedentary existence. Such restriction of exercise, however, leads to deconditioning which may adversely affect exercise tolerance. Therefore, patients with heart failure should be advised to maintain exercise levels within their exercise capacity. Isotonic exercises like walking or bicycling are preferred to isometric exercise.

Drugs

Diuretics decrease preload and hence alleviate systemic and pulmonary venous congestion.

Vasodilators are probably the most useful addition to the treatment of DCM. ACE inhibitors and a combination of isosorbide dinitrate and hydralazine not only control symptoms and improve effort tolerance, but most importantly prolong life. They should be the firstline of drug therapy in patients with DCM.

Digoxin has been shown to be effective in patients with severe cardiac failure. A number of newer inotropic agents have been tried and have been shown to improve hemodynamics and symptoms during short-term management. None of these has been shown to prolong life.

Beta blockers act by decreasing myocardial oxygen consumption, decreasing deleterious effects of catecholamines, upregulating myocardial beta receptors, improving diastolic function of the myocardium. Trials to evaluate the efficacy of these drugs are in progress, and these drugs should be considered only after serious deliberation because of their negative inotropic effect.

A majority of patients of DCM die suddenly due to arrhythmias. Although drugs like amiodarone have been shown to decrease the incidence of these arrhythmias, their effect on prognosis is not clear.

Immunosuppressive therapy: A subset of patients of DCM (especially those with a history of less than 6 months' duration) show myocardial histology simulating myocarditis. Immunosuppressive drugs including steroids, azathioprine and cyclosporine may improve hemodynamics, symptoms and prognosis in this subset of patients.

Anticoagulants: There is a high incidence of thrombus formation in the cardiac chambers and in the deep veins of the legs with systemic and pulmonary embolism. Long-term anticoagulant therapy should be used in patients who have had episodes of embolism or have a thrombus in the cardiac chambers on echocardiography or whose LV size is large.

Cardiac Transplantation
This is reserved for those who are terminally sick and have a life expectancy of less than 6 months.

Prognosis

The following features are indicative of poor prognosis
1. Age above 55 years or less than 10 years
2. Left ventricular conduction delay
3. Absence of left ventricular hypertrophy
4. Cardiothoracic ratio greater than 55 percent
5. Cardiac index less than 2.6 liters/min/m^2

Alcoholic Cardiomyopathy

Alcoholic cardiomyopathy is the commonest type of secondary cardiomyopathy. The reported incidence of 5–10 percent is probably an understatement. It is important to elicit history of prolonged alcohol abuse from every patient with cardiomyopathy irrespective of age, sex, social class or cultural background. Alcohol causes deleterious effect on the myocardium by three mechanisms:
a. Direct toxic effect of alcohol or its metabolites
b. Autoimmune mechanism
c. Nutritional deficiency, especially of thiamine.

Alcoholic cardiomyopathy is reversible, at least initially, if the patients stop taking alcohol. On the other hand, if the patient continues to drink, mortality is around 80 percent in three years. Alcoholic cardiomyopathy should be differentiated from "holiday heart syndrome" which is characterized by supraventricular (mainly atrial fibrillation) and occasionally ventricular arrhythmias after an alcoholic binge.

Restrictive Cardiomyopathy

This is the least common type of cardiomyopathy. The primary abnormality is abnormal ventricular diastolic function (decreased compliance) with normal to near-normal systolic function (contractility) and normal ventricular internal dimensions.

The restrictive cardiomyopathy (RCM) is diagnosed by demonstration of elevation in left and right ventricular filling pressures (raised LVEDP and RVEDP). In contrast to normal persons, in RCM, ventricular filling is accomplished almost entirely during early diastole.

Diastolic ventricular function may be primarily impaired in the absence of morphologically detectable myocardial or endomyocardial disease (idiopathic RCM) (Table 7.2).

The clinical presentation of chronic constrictive pericarditis (CCP) closely simulates that of RCM. It is of paramount importance to differentiate CCP from RCM because CCP is a surgically curable condition while RCM is an essentially progressive disorder with no known modality of treatment.

Table 7.2: Classification of RCM

Myocardial		
A.	Noninfiltrative diseases	
	Idiopathic	
	Scleroderma	
B.	Infiltrative diseases	
	Amyloid	
	Sarcoid	
	Gaucher's disease	
	Hurler's disease	
C.	Storage diseases	
	Hemochromatosis	
	Fabry's disease	
	Glycogen storage disease	
Endomyocardial		
	Endomyocardial fibrosis	
	Hypereosinophilic syndrome	
	Carcinoid	
	Metastatic malignancies	
	Radiation	
	Anthracycline toxicity (rare)	

Clinical Features

History: Symptoms of marked pulmonary venous congestion and chest pain, especially anginal, favor RCM. History suggestive of tuberculosis elsewhere in the body and past history of pericardiocentesis favor CCP.

Clinical examination: A well-defined left ventricular type of apex beat, paradoxically split S_2, murmurs of atrioventricular valve regurgitation and significant pulmonary hypertension (loud P2 which is palpable) favor RCM.

Investigations

Chest X-ray: Significant pulmonary venous hypertension and pulmonary edema favor a diagnosis of RCM. Pericardial calcification on anteroposterior and lateral penetrated chest X-ray and on fluoroscopy is strongly suggestive of a diagnosis of CCP.

Echocardiography: Pericardial thickening and calcification and Doppler echocardiography of atrioventricular valves and hepatic veins have also been found to be useful in differentiating RCM from CCP.

ECG: Evidence of ventricular hypertrophy, LBBB or intraventricular conduction defects, pattern simulating large myocardial infarction (large Q waves, poor progression of precordial R waves), complete heart block or other bradyarrhythmias, and atrial fibrillation (rare in CCP) favor a diagnosis of RCM.

CT scan can detect minute amounts of pericardial calcification. It is also very specific for detecting pericardial thickening. MRI may be useful in differentiating RCM and CCP. Endomyocardial biopsy may be of great help in certain infiltrative disorders of the heart that present as RCM.

Prognosis

The clinical course of idiopathic RCM may be protracted and prolonged survival is not uncommon.

Management

There is no known treatment for RCM. Digoxin in useful in atrial fibrillation while in sinus rhythm it is of no use. Calcium-channel blockers may improve diastolic function but their role in improving symptoms or long-term course is yet to be documented. In high-grade AV block, permanent pacemaker is usually required. Genetic counseling is important as idiopathic RCM is occasionally familial.

Congenital Heart Disease

The incidence of congenital heart disease (CHD) is about 1:100 livebirths. In premature babies there is high incidence of patent ductus arteriosus (PDA), and 4 times the incidence of ventricular septal defect (VSD). In small for birth babies again there is a high incidence of PDA, VSD, atrial septal defect (ASD), and tetralogy of Fallot (TOF). In babies of diabetic mothers there is 5–10 times more incidence of VSD, aortic malformations and transposition of great vessels (TGV). Following a birth of a child with CHD, the recurrence rate in a second child is 2 percent. In adults one can come across ASD, VSD, PDA, tetralogy of Fallot and Eisenmenger's syndrome. Nowadays almost all defects are diagnosed and treated in childhood.

Etiology

The etiology is genetic in 8 percent, environmental in 2 percent and multifactorial in 90 percent.

Genetic causes are gene defects or chromosomal abnormalities.

Environmental factors include maternal diabetes, rubella or other infections during pregnancy in the mother, intake of drugs during pregnancy (thalidomide, trimethadione, etc.), excessive maternal alcohol consumption, and maternal diabetes mellitus and systemic lupus erythematosus.

Clinical Features

The common clinical features of all CHD will be discussed here. The other characteristics of individual defects will be mentioned later on.

The child is brought with the parents complaining of failure to thrive, difficulty in feeding, tachycardia, tachypnea, excessive sweating and cardiomegaly. At times a murmur is detected on routine auscultation after birth or during vaccination.

The mother may note blue discoloration of nails and tongue especially when the child cries.

With obstructive lesions like AS, there may be fatigue and tiredness in an older child, or even angina and syncope. There is a risk of sudden cardiac death also. Sometimes tachycardia in ASD or AV block in TGV brings the child to attention. Sometimes tachycardia in ASD or AV block in TGV brings the child to attention. Cerebral abscess is a common complication and a presenting feature of CHD with right to left shunts. In Eisenmenger's syndrome there may be right sided failure. Clotting abnormalities can occur in cyanotic CHD due to polycythemia (Table 8.1).

Diagnosis

Presence of cyanosis differentiates between cyanotic and acyanotic diseases. Clubbing is seen in cyanotics. X-ray, ECG and echocardiogram is usually sufficient for diagnosis. Cardiac catheterization may be required in complex heart disease before surgery.

Treatment

Most cases will require surgery. Surgery may be curative or palliative. Failure is treated in usual way.

Atrial Septal Defect

ASD constitutes 15 percent of all CHD and is commoner in females (Fig. 8.1).

Table 8.1: Common congenital heart diseases

	Neonate	Infant and older child
Cyanotic	TGA	TOF, TGA
	Tricuspid atresia	
	Severe PS, pulmonary atresia	
	Severe Ebstein with ASD	
Acyanotic	Congenital AS	VSD, ASD, PDA
	Coarctation of aorta	AS, coarctation, PS, PAPVC

Types

1. Secundum: commonest—80 percent
2. Primum: 15 percent
3. Sinus venosus.

Formation

In the fetus from 5th week, the septum primum develops from the roof of atrium and divides the fetal common atrium goes toward the endocardial cushion. The foramen primum occurs at the junction of the septum primum and the endocardial cushion. A second septum develops similarly and at the top the foramen secundum is formed when the foramen primum closes. If the foramen primum remains open it is called the primum defect and if the foramen secundum remains patent it is called the secundum defect. In sinus venosus defect the ASD occurs at the junction of SVC or IVC to RA. The blood can flow from SVC or IVC to LA.

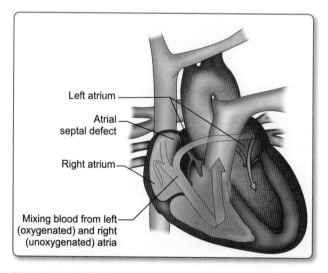

Fig. 8.1: Atrial septal defect

Pathophysiology

The foramina allow fetal circulation to complete as the oxygenation occurs in placenta and the oxygenated blood reaches RA. Then it crosses the ASD to LA and LV and all parts of body. If this foramen remains open after birth, the blood flows from LA to RA as RV has lesser compliance. As a result RA, RV and PA receive double the blood. The pulmonary vasculature reacts to this increased flow by increasing its resistance. So pulmonary hypertension, RVH and later on right heart failure develops (Eisenmenger's syndrome).

Clinical Presentation

Most patients of ASD are asymptomatic in childhood and may be diagnosed in 3rd or 4th decade. They may have recurrent respiratory infection, mild effort intolerance and 1 vague left sided chest pains. Later in life they present with heart failure or arrhythmias.

The JVP may be raised and 'a' and 'v' waves are equal. A precordial heave may be felt due to RV overload. The sinequa non of ASD is a fixed splitting of S_2 with loss of respiratory variation. This is because the ASD distributes blood equally to LA and RA during inspiration and due to volume overload the P_2 is late. P_2 may be loud. A systolic murmur grade 2–3 is best heard in left 2nd or 3rd space due to increased flow across the pulmonary valve. A mitral regurgitant murmur is heard in primum defects due to a cleft mitral or tricuspid valve. A tricuspid diastolic murmur is heard with large left to right shunts. When pulmonary hypertension develops there is a soft ejection systolic murmur, an ejection click, a loud P_2 and TR murmur disappears. MVP is often associated.

ECG: Right axis and an incomplete RBBB are seen. In primum defect a left axis with LAHB.

X-ray chest will show cardiomegaly of RV type, increased rightward convexity due to right atrial enlargement a prominent PA, increased vascularity of lungs (pulmonary plethora). On screening this is seen as 'hilar dance'. If pulmonary vascular obstructive disease develops, the main pulmonary artery is quite large and peripheral lung fields become oligemic (Fig. 8.2).

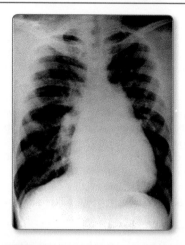

Fig. 8.2: X-ray chest in atrial septal defect

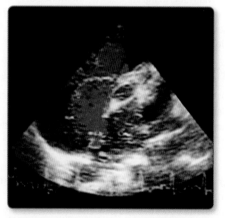

Fig. 8.3: Echocardiography in atrial septal defect

Echocardiogram: It shows enlarged RA, RV. The septal defect is visualized, flow across is documented with Doppler or contract echocardiography and associated MVP, MR or TR seen. It also allows measurement of the size of the defect. IVS moves paradoxically (moving away from lateral LV wall in systole). Pulmonary pressures can be estimated (Fig. 8.3).

Treatment

Closure of ASD is recommended when the pulmonary to systemic flow is above 1.5:1 especially when RV size is increased. The optimum age is between 4 and 5 years the aim is to prevent pulmonary hypertension in the young and atrial arrhythmias and failure in the older patients. There is a survival benefit for patients older than 50 years also even if they are asymptomatic. Surgical treatment is contraindicated in patients with pulmonary arterial hypertension and right-to-left shunt.

It can be done with a device in catheterization laboratory in suitable patients or by surgery.

Secundum ASD does not require endocarditis prophylaxis but primum ASD or associated MVP will require the prophylaxis.

Patent Foramen Ovale

About 25 percent have incomplete closure of foramen ovale at birth. Normally it is insignificant. The incidence of PFO is higher in patients with cryptogenic stroke. Closing them with devices decreased the stroke incidence. It is speculated that PFO also is associated with migraine.

Ventricular Septal Defect

The VSD is the commonest congenital heart defect, occurring in 25–30 percent of patients with CHD or 2 perlive births. It affects both sexes equally. It is often associated with other defects of the heart (Fig. 8.4).

Types

1. Perimembranous: occurring in 80 percent makes it the commonest type.
2. Muscular: It occurs in 5–20 percent. Subdivided into central, apical, marginal and Swiss cheese types.
3. Inlet VSD
4. Outlet VSD. 5–7 percent, occurs below the pulmonary valve.

Pathophysiology

The VSD causes the oxygenated blood to flow from LV to RV at a high pressure gradient throughout the systole. Most of the

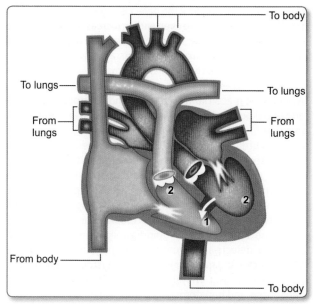

Fig. 8.4: Ventricular septal defect; 1. Hole or defect in ventricular septum; 2. Ventricles

blood is shunted directed to PA without causing RV volume overload. PA pressure increases as it receives blood from both RV and LV. The lungs become plethoric. The flow reaches LA and the excess flow across MV causes a functional middiastolic murmur. The LV ejects into both major arteries and so the systole is shortened, the aortic valve closes early resulting in a moderately wide split S_2. The hemodynamics depend on the size of VSD, the pulmonary vascular resistance and presence of other defects like PS. A VSD less than half the aortic orifice will cause a small left to right shunt. If both are of equal size the pressures in both ventricles will be equalized. If PVR is normal the left to right shunt is high, with high PVR the shunt is small.

Clinical Features

Infants with VSD become symptomatic at the age of 6–10 weeks, when the pulmonary vascular resistance falls to normal levels, and develop heart failure if the defect is large. Premature babies may develop heart failure even earlier; increased sweating due to increased sympathetic tone, fatigue, dyspnea during feeding and recurrent respiratory infections and retarded growth chronic ill health are the main symptoms.

On physical examination, there is a wide pulse pressure, hyperkinetic precordium with bulge and a systolic thrill at the left sternal border. The heart is enlarged with a left ventricular apex. The first and second heart sounds are masked by the pan systolic murmur at the lower left sternal border. At the second left interspace, the second sound is normally split with small left-to-right shunts, but is widely split and variable with large shunts. In patients with pulmonary arterial hypertension the second sound is closely split or may even be single. With a small to moderate sized shunt a third heart sound is heard at the apex. With large shunts an apical middiastolic murmur is present. With large defects and equalization of pressure between the two ventricles, the murmur loses its pan systolic character and is audible as an ejection systolic murmur. There will be bilateral crepitations and hepatomegaly in case of failure.

Spontaneous closure occurs in 30–50 percent of small defects. It is common in defects in muscular or membranous part.

Complications: AR in 5 percent, endocarditis, infundibular stenosis and pulmonary hypertension.

Investigations

ECG: It will show biventricular hypertrophy (45 mm voltage in midprecordial leads: Katz-Wachtel phenomenon). There is left axis deviation. ECG may be normal in small VSD.

X-ray chest: In small VSD the cardiac size is normal. In others the cardiac size is enlarged and the pulmonary vasculature is prominent. In large shunts LA and main PA are also enlarged (Fig. 8.5).

If severe pulmonary resistance sets in the main pulmonary artery is very prominent and the vasculature is reduced in outer 1/3rd of the lung fields.

Echocardiography: Echo with color Doppler can detect the location, size and shunt across the defect. The size is considered in respect of

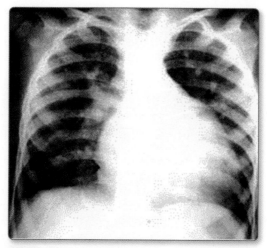

Fig. 8.5: X-ray chest in ventricular septal defect

aortic root size: A defect equal to bigger than aortic route is termed large VSD, one equal to half or 2/3rd is moderate and if less than 1/3rd aortic dimension is considered small (Fig. 8.6).

Cardiac catheterization is done to define the anatomic defect and also for associated anomalies. It shows step up of oxygen saturation in RV.

Management

For patients with small VSD no specific therapy is needed except for infective endocarditis prophylaxis. Failure is managed with diuretics, ACE inhibitors and digoxin. The indications for surgery are as follows: Large defects (> 1 cm/m^2, shunt > 2:1, increasing heart size on X-ray chest), increasing AR, previous endocarditis, Increased PVR may result in Eisenmenger's complex at 10–15 years of age.

Device closure is possible for muscular VSDs but not for the membranous VSD.

Surgical closure of VSD is done before 3 years of age and earlier if medical management fails to relieve symptoms. Patients with large VSD and left-to-right shunt larger than 1.5:1 with PVR/SVR ratio of 0.5 and PVR less than 7 Wood units/m^2

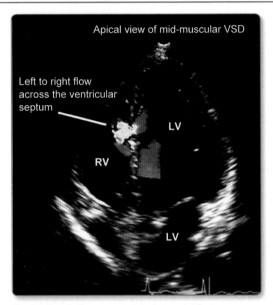

Apical view of mid-muscular VSD

Left to right flow across the ventricular septum

LV

RV

LV

Fig. 8.6: Doppler flow across ventricular septal defect

should be operated on. It can be done in infancy and newborns also if failure is gross.

Patent Ductus Arteriosus

The ductus normally closes functionally within 24–48 hours after birth. Premature babies commonly have persistent ductus arteriosus which closes spontaneously when the baby reaches the full-term age.

The patent ductus arteriosus (PDA) accounts for about 10 percent of congenital heart diseases. It is slightly more common in females and is the commonest congenital lesion in babies with rubella syndrome. Babies born at high altitude have a higher incidence. 50 percent of premature babies have patent PDA.

Pathophysiology

The PDA results in a left-to-right shunt from the aorta to the pulmonary artery throughout the cardiac cycle as the aortic pressure is higher than the pulmonary artery pressure both in systole as well as in diastole. This results in a continuous murmur. The pulmonary arteries receive the flow through the PDA as well as the right ventricle. The large flow passing through a normal mitral valve results in a mitral middiastolic murmur. The left ventricle receives an increased volume of blood in diastole and thereby enlarges in size. The systolic ejection phase of the left ventricle is prolonged, causing a delayed closure of the aortic valve. The large flow passes through the ascending aorta and the arch, resulting in their enlargement. The enlarged aorta results in a constant ejection click.

Patients are asymptomatic and the PDA is detected during school medical exam. Large shunts can cause symptoms of LVF. Later on pulmonary hypertension develops and when it is more than systemic pressure there is a reversal of shunt (Eisenmenger's syndrome). The patient will have pink fingers and blue toes as the pulmonary arterial blood goes preferentially downwards.

Clinical Features

The PDA is usually asymptomatic. There may be repeated chest infections and failure to thrive. Older children may complain of dyspnea and palpitations.

The pulse pressure is wide with a bounding character (feel the foot pulses in babies). The precordium is hyperactive with pulsations in suprasternal notch and prominent carotid pulsations. Cardiac apex is of LV type with a hyperkinetic impulse. A systolic or continuous thrill may be palpable in left 2nd space especially in thin persons. S_1 is loud and S_2 is split normally in small shunts and is single or paradoxically split in large ones. A continuous 'machinery' murmur can be heard below the left clavicle and this can mask S_2. A third sound is heard at apex with small shunts and a middiastolic rumble in large shunts.

With development of pulmonary hypertension, diastolic component disappears and systolic component becomes shorter and with an ejection quality. P_2 is loud. S_2 is single or is reversed. Sometimes dilatation of PA results in pulmonary regurgitation. VSD, PS, coarctation may be associated.

Investigations

ECG shows LVH and normal axis.

X-ray chest shows cardiomegaly with prominent LV configuration, and LA enlargement. The man pulmonary artery and pulmonary arterial markings are increased. Ascending aorta is prominent.

Echocardiography

This will show the site of shunt and Doppler will quantify the shunt.

Catheterization

This is done if additional lesions are suspected. The pulmonary arterial oxygen saturation is higher than that in the right ventricle. Right atrial pressure is normal. The pulmonary arterial pressure is normal with a small PDA and a small left-to-right shunt, while it is increased with large shunt; pulmonary arterial wedge pressure may be increased with large shunt. Passage of the cardiac catheter from the pulmonary artery to the descending aorta during the study proves the presence of the ductus arteriosus (Fig. 8.7).

An aortic angiogram in the left anterior oblique view identifies the PDA and also excludes aortopulmonary septal defect.

Treatment

If the PDA is identified within the first 2 weeks of life, medical closure using indomethacin (0.2 mg/kg 12 hourly for 3 doses) can be attempted. The treatment is contraindicated in the presence of jaundice or renal insufficiency. Medical treatment consists of control of chest infections and treatment of heart failure.

Nonsurgical closure is done with occluder devices like Rashkind umbrella or coils. Surgical closure can be done safely after age of 3 months and should preferably be done in preschool years. Preferably it should be divided rather than ligated so the recanalization won't occur. Surgery is contraindicated in presence of right to left shunt.

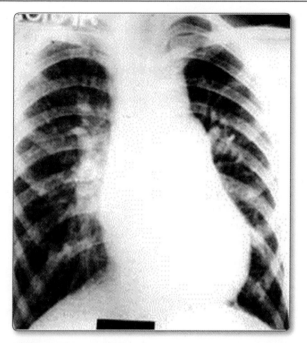

Fig. 8.7: X-ray in patent ductus arteriosus

Course and Prognosis

The problems are development of pulmonary hypertension and endocarditis, the later occurs on the pulmonary artery opposite the ductus.

Tetralogy of Fallot

Fallot in 1888 described a combination of four defects: Ventricular septal defect, right ventricular outflow tract (RVOT) obstruction, overriding of aorta and hypertrophy of right ventricle. Tetralogy of Fallot (TOF) accounts for 10–15 percent of all CHD. The sex distribution is equal or shows a slight male predominance. It is the commonest cyanotic heart disease after 1 year of age (Table 8.2).

Table 8.2: Cyanotic congenital heart disease classification

A.	Increased pulmonary arterial blood flow	
	1.	Transposition of great arteries
	2.	Truncus arteriosus
	3.	Total anomalous pulmonary venous connection (TAPVC)
	4.	Single ventricle without pulmonary stenosis
B.	Normal or decreased pulmonary arterial blood flow	
	1. Dominant left ventricle	
		A. Tricuspid atresia
		B. Pulmonary atresia with intact ventricular septum
		C. Ebstein's anomaly of tricuspid valve
	2. Dominant right ventricle without pulmonary hypertension	
		A. Tetralogy of Fallot
		B. Pulmonary stenosis with right-to-left shunt at atrial level
		C. Double-outlet right ventricle
		D. Transposition of great arteries with pulmonary stenosis

Pathophysiology

Since the VSD is large, the pressures in the right and left ventricles are identical. The magnitude of right-to-left shunt is determined by the resistance offered at the systemic and pulmonary vascular levels; since the resistance to right ventricular outflow exceeds the systemic level, the shunt is right to left.

Clinical Features

Cyanosis is rare at birth, but is noticed usually at the end of the first year; it may be more obvious on effort such as crying, feeding and coughing. Hypoxic spells occur in about 20 percent of patients. These spells are initiated by feeding, crying or waking up from sleep, and are characterized by tachypnea, increasing cyanosis, syncope and occasionally convulsions. They appear in infancy and are rare after the age of two.

Squatting after exertion is the other common feature. This increases SVR and reduces right-to-left shunt and increases pulmonary flow.

There is secondary polycythemia and may result in arterial or venous thrombosis, particularly cerebral. There can be cerebral abscess due to the absence of lung filter with right-to-left shunt, infective endocarditis and paradoxical embolism (Fig. 8.8).

Physical Examination

There is a variable degree of physical underdevelopment; central cyanosis and clubbing are present (Fig. 8.9). The precordial impulse is quiet with no evidence of cardiomegaly. A_2 may be palpable. There is an ejection systolic murmur best heard in the 3rd left intercostal space. The murmur originates in the infundibular stenosis and varies inversely with the severity of obstruction and is not due to VSD. The 2nd sound is loud and single with only the aortic component being heard. Continuous murmur due to collaterals through the bronchial arteries is sometimes heard in the paravertebral area.

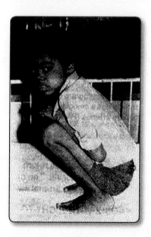

Fig. 8.8: The squatting posture often seen in tetralogy of Fallot

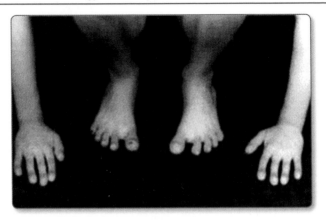

Fig. 8.9: Clubbing and toes and finger nails

Investigations

X-ray chest: Classically heart shape is of coeur en sabot (heart in a boot) appearance with apex lifted off the left hemidiaphragm by RVH. In the usual site of PA there is concavity. Lung fields are oligemic. Aortic knuckle is good sized and may be right sided in 25 percent of cases.

The ECG shows right axis deviation, right ventricular hypertrophy with incomplete or complete RBBB, with an early transitional zone in V_2 or V_3. VPCs are common as also paroxysmal ventricular tachycardia.

Echocardiography permits visualization of the VSD, overriding of aorta and the narrowed RVOT. Doppler studies identify the site of right-to-left shunt and any other associated valvular abnormality.

Cardiac catheterization and angiocardiography give the anatomical details such as the architecture of RVOT, the size of the pulmonary arteries, the degree of overriding and the size of the left ventricle.

Course and Prognosis

Two-thirds of patients with TOF reach the age of 3 years; only 25 percent complete their first decade of life without surgical treatment. The commonest causes of death are cyanotic spells, cerebral abscess, and cerebral thrombosis due to polycythemia, infective endocarditis and rarely congestive heart failure.

Management

Cyanotic spells are treated by placing the child in the knee-chest position and administering oxygen and subcutaneous morphine 0.2 mg/kg weight. If there is acidosis, sodabicarb is required. Vasopressors, beta-blockers and general anesthesia may be needed in resistant cases. Propranolol is useful for prevention of spells. The recommended dose is 1–4 mg/kg body weight/24 hours given orally. Avoid dehydration which can increase polycythemia.

Surgical Management

1. If the child is asymptomatic or minimally symptomatic, intracardiac repair is recommended between 18 and 36 months of age.
2. Children below this age who are symptomatic or whose spells are not controlled with propranolol can undergo intracardiac repair or a shunt surgery. Shunt surgery consists of improving the pulmonary blood flow by creating a channel between the subclavian and the pulmonary arteries (Blalock-Taussig shunt), or between the ascending aorta and pulmonary artery (Waterston Cooley shunt). Later total correction can be done at about 2 years of age. The intracardiac repair carries a mortality of 5 percent. The VSD is closed by a dacron patch, and the infundibular stenosis is relieved by excising the muscle bundles. Sometimes, the RVOT is enlarged by using a pericardial patch. Surgical results have improved with better techniques and technology of open-heart surgery.

Transposition of Great Arteries (Complete Transposition, D-transposition)

Transposition means that the aorta arises from the right ventricle and pulmonary artery from the left ventricle. The aorta lies anterior and to the right of pulmonary artery (d-loop). This accounts for about 10 percent of cyanotic heart diseases. The male: female ratio is 4:1. The systemic and pulmonary circulations function in parallel rather than series. Survival depends on mixing between systemic and pulmonary circulations at the atrial, ventricular or aortopulmonary level (Fig. 8.10).

Clinical features consist of signs of heart failure developing within 2–6 weeks of life. The child is cyanotic at birth (as compared to TOF). The electrocardiogram shows right axis deviation, right ventricular hypertrophy, and right atrial overload.

The diagnostic triad on chest X-ray includes oval or egg-shaped cardiac contour, moderate cardiomegaly and increased pulmonary vascular markings.

The diagnosis is confirmed by echocardiography and cardiac catheterization with angiocardiography, echocardiography is diagnostic. The anterior aorta and posterior PA are seen. Additional defects like ASD, VSD, LVOTO or PDA may be seen.

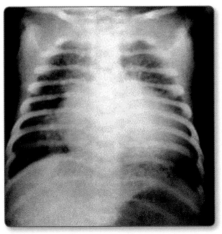

Fig. 8.10: X-ray of transposition of great arteries

Without treatment 30 percent of these infants die in the first week and 90 percent within the first year. Creation of an atrial septal defect by balloon atrial septostomy or by surgery is useful in hypoxic children, by allowing better mixing of blood in the cardiac chambers. In cyanotic infants whose pulmonary blood flow is dependent on a patent ductus arteriosus the latency of the latter can be maintained by prostaglandin E_1 infusion (0.05 to 1 μg/kg/min). This is a major help in stabilizing the infant while other procedures are being planned (Fig. 8.11).

In the intraatrial repair the venous return is redirected to respective ventricles at the atrial level. (Senning or Mustard procedure). The operation that is gaining more popularity is now the arterial switch operation (switching the arteries to their respective ventricles).

Corrected Transposition (L-transposition)

The aorta lies anterior and to the left of pulmonary artery (d-loop).Transposition means that the aorta arises from the anatomical right ventricle but present in LV position and

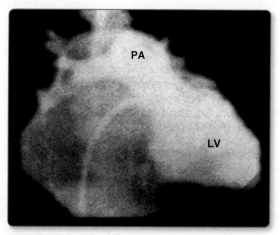

Fig. 8.11: Left ventricular angiogram of a child with transposition. This ventricle has a smooth configuration and gives rise to pulmonary arteries (PA = pulmonary artery; LV = left ventricle)

pulmonary artery from the morphological left ventricle but present in RV position. Thus circulation occurs in normal fashion. But associated lesions cause morbidity. They are VSD (in 70–90 percent), PS (in 40 percent), AR, complete AV block. Features and treatment are of the associated defect.

Total Anomalous Pulmonary Venous Connection (TAPVC)

The entire pulmonary venous blood drains directly or indirectly into the right atrium, leading to a large left-to-right shunt. There is usually an intertribal right-to-left communication, as the only source for the left atrium. Development of pulmonary hypertension is common with pulmonary venous obstruction. As the pulmonary vascular resistance increases, the pulmonary flow decreases, resulting in marked systemic arterial desaturation.

Clinical Features

Cyanosis and clubbing are partly related to the presence and severity of pulmonary venous obstruction. There may be evidence of congestive cardiac failure in about one-third of patients. Other patients have features of a large atrial septal defect. A prominent left precordium, hyperdynamic right ventricular impulse, and wide and fixed splitting of second sound are present. An ejection systolic murmur is heard at the upper left sternal border and a loud middiastolic flow murmur is audible in the tricuspid area.

Electrocardiogram shows right axis deviation, tall peaked P waves, right ventricular hypertrophy and RBBB.

Chest X-ray reveals cardiac enlargement, prominent right atrium, prominent main pulmonary artery segment and pulmonary plethora. In the supracardiac variety, the confluence of pulmonary veins drains into the left innominate or superior vena cava, resulting in the distinctive "figure of eight" or "snow-man in snowstorm" or 'cottage loaf' appearance (Fig. 8.12).

Almost 75 percent to 90 percent of infants die in the first year. The prognosis is worse if associated with pulmonary

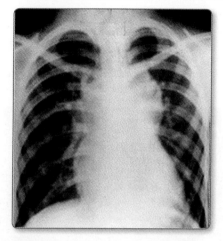

Fig. 8.12: X-ray of total anomalous pulmonary venous connection

venous obstruction and is better in patients with a large atrial septal defect. A balloon atrial septostomy may be life-saving in critically ill neonates. In uncomplicated cases, complete repair of the defect is possible after one year of age, with an overall mortality of 10 percent.

Ebstein's Anomaly

Ebstein's anomaly refers to a downward displacement of tricuspid valve tissue into the right ventricle. Thus, a portion of the right ventricle acts like a right atrium. This atrialized right ventricle contracts poorly and interferes with right ventricular filling.

Dyspnea, fatigue and palpitations are the usual symptoms. Cyanosis is present due to right-to-left shunt at the atrial level. A systolic murmur of tricuspid regurgitation is heard at the lower left sternal border. The first and 2nd heart sounds are widely split, and 3rd and 4th heart sounds may be heard. Thus, multiple heart sounds are an important feature of Ebstein's anomaly (Fig. 8.13).

Box-like globular cardiac configuration is seen on chest X-ray, which closely resembles a large pericardial effusion. ECG shows tall and peaked P waves, often referred to as Himalayan. The diagnosis is confirmed by echocardiography (Fig. 8.14).

The tricuspid valve is displaced into the right ventricle and that part of the right ventricle behaves like the right atrium

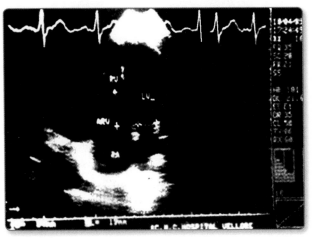

Fig. 8.13: Echocardiographic picture of a patient with Ebstein's anomaly

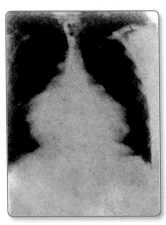

Fig. 8.14: Chest X-ray of 4-year-old child with Ebstein's anomaly. There is marked cardiomegaly with right atrial enlargement

and is called atrialized right ventricle (ARV). In this case, the displacement was 34 mm when compared with the mitral annulus.

Patients who are symptomatic should undergo a tricuspid valve repair in which marsupialization of the atrialized right ventricle is undertaken with realignment of the tricuspid cusps to the tricuspid annulus. This procedure is preferred over operations in which the tricuspid valve is replaced with a prosthetic valve.

Eisenmenger Syndrome

The term Eisenmenger syndrome is used if there is severe pulmonary hypertension in patients with atrial or ventricular septal defects or patent ductus arteriosus resulting in reversal of the left-to-right shunt. The pulmonary arterial pressures are equal to or higher than the systemic arterial pressure. This disorder accounts for about 7 percent of adult CHD, and is more common in females. The term Eisenmenger complex is used if the shunt is at the ventricular level.

Clinical Features

Dyspnea is the main symptom. Hemoptysis, chest pain and fainting attacks are common in adolescence or later in life. Cyanosis and clubbing are present. If the reversal of the shunt is at the ductus level, it is associates with a 'differential' cyanosis, i.e. cyanosis is noted only in the lower limbs. (Fig. 8.15).

A parasternal heave is present. The second sound is loud and single, or split with P_2 component being very loud. There is often an early diastolic murmur due to pulmonary regurgitation.

Investigations

Chest X-ray: The main pulmonary artery and its main branches are dilated and prominent. The peripheral vessels are difficult to make out.

Electrocardiogram: There is severe right ventricular hypertrophy.

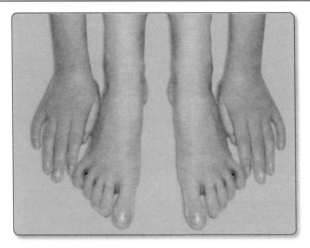

Fig. 8.15: Differential cyanosis

Course and Prognosis

The course is invariably progressive and complications related to progressive polycythemia, pulmonary infarction or hemoptysis occur. Only a few patients survive beyond 40 years.

Management

Surgical closure of the defects is contraindicated in this disorder as this will result in severe right ventricular failure and death. These patients are treated symptomatically with drugs for managing congestive heart failure. Heart lung transplant may be the only recourse.

Pregnancy and Heart Disease

Any heart disease which can develop in a nonpregnant woman can occur in a pregnant woman. In addition, pregnancy may produce diseases or modifications of diseases which are peculiar to pregnancy itself.

Hemodynamics of Normal Pregnancy

In a normal pregnancy there is a 40 percent increase in maternal blood volume and cardiac output. The increase in blood volume is by about 40 percent and is mainly attributed to estrogen-mediated stimulation of rennin. Heart rate: The rise in heart rate peaks during the third trimester. The average rise in heart rate is 10–20 beats per minute. Vasodilatation leads to decline in PVR and diastolic blood pressure. Pulse pressure increases. These changes peak during 2nd trimester.

Hemodynamic changes during labor and delivery: Cardiac output increases by up to 50 percent during uterine contractions mainly due to changes in stroke volume. Both systolic and diastolic blood pressures increase markedly during the second stage.

Postpartum changes: Venous return increases after delivery of the fetus and relief from the caval compression. In addition, blood shifting from the contracting, emptied uterus into the systemic circulation increases the preload. The increase in effective blood volume occurs despite blood loss associated with delivery and leads to substantial rise in stroke volume and cardiac output immediately after delivery. Within the first hour, however, the reduction in heart rate decreases cardiac output, which falls to prepregnancy levels by 24 hours postpartum as stroke volume normalizes.

Clinical Features

Cardiac examination in a normal pregnant woman may sound like a washing machine. With volume overload and rapid filling of LV there can be an S_3 gallop. A murmur is common due to high flow across pulmonary valve. A bruit for the breast may be confused. Murmurs from stenotic lesions become louder. The physical findings of MVP or IHSS may disappear with increased LV volume.

Course

There is a high risk of maternal mortality in Eisenmenger's syndrome, pulmonary hypertension, (> 50 mmHg), Marfan's syndrome with dilated aortic root and history of peripartum cardiomyopathy. These conditions are also considered contraindications for pregnancy and are indications for termination of pregnancy. The risk is moderate in NYHA class III or IV MS, AS, Marfan's syndrome with normal aortic root, uncomplicated coarctation and previous MI. The risk is low with septal defects, PDA, pulmonic and tricuspid valve lesions and NYHA class I and II.

Mitral stenosis is the most commonly encountered rheumatic valvular lesion in pregnancy (Fig. 9.1). The physiologic increase in cardiac output and heart rate results in significant increase in the resting pressure gradient in the second trimester of pregnancy. The arrhythmogenic effect of pregnancy may result in atrial flutter or fibrillation, substantially accelerating the ventricular rate and further elevating left atrial pressure. In addition to the decreased serum colloid osmotic pressure, often a result of peripartum intravenous fluid administration, these changes predispose to pulmonary edema during the peripartum period.

Therapeutic abortion should be considered in patients with pulmonary hypertension or NYHA class III or IV symptoms during the first trimester. In patients with class I or II symptoms, medical line of treatment should be followed. This consists of bed rest, salt restriction, diuretics, beta-blockers, prompt treatment of infections and correction of anemia.

In patients with significant mitral stenosis (mitral valve area < 1.5 cm^2) and more than class II symptoms despite adequate medical therapy, consideration should be given to either balloon mitral valvuloplasty (BMV) or surgical intervention. Surgery does not seem to affect maternal mortality, but fetal mortality is approximately 10 percent and surgery in early

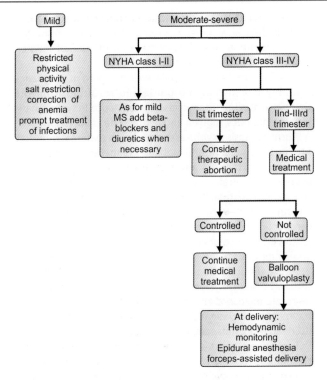

Fig. 9.1: Management of mitral stenosis in pregnancy

pregnancy may be associated with abortion later in pregnancy and premature labor. Hence, BMV may have an edge over surgery, provided that it is done in later stages of pregnancy to avoid the teratogenic effects of radiation during the period of organogenesis.

In symptomatic patients or those with moderate or severe stenosis, hemodynamic monitoring with a pulmonary artery catheter is recommended during labor, delivery and puerperium. Epidural anesthesia is recommended and is often associated with significant fall in pulmonary arterial and left atrial pressures owing to systemic vasodilation. Forceps-assisted delivery should be considered to circumvent the repeated prolonged Valsalva maneuvers required for vaginal delivery.

The patients are advised to restrict the number of children to one or two and undergo tubal ligation.

Mitral regurgitation is usually well-tolerated in pregnancy probably because of the unloading resulting from the physiological fall in systemic vascular resistance. In symptomatic patients, diuretics, digoxin and hydralazine are of help.

Aortic stenosis may be associated with maternal mortality rates up to 17 percent, and high rates of therapeutic abortions and fetal mortality. If aortic stenosis is diagnosed before pregnancy, surgical correction before conception is advisable. In a patient with aortic stenosis who is already pregnant, measures to prevent hypovolemia and to restrict activity are appropriate. If symptoms are progressive and cannot be controlled with standard medical management, aortic valve surgery or aortic balloon valvulotomy should be performed.

Aortic regurgitation is well-tolerated during pregnancy probably because systemic vascular resistance is reduced and heart rate increased and thus diastolic filling time is reduced. In symptomatic patients, diuretics, digoxin and hydralazine for afterload reduction can be safely used.

Even open heart surgery can be performed with due precautions.

Arrhythmias may develop or worsen during pregnancy. With most preexisting arrhythmias pregnancy is well-tolerated. Look for correctable causes like electrolyte disturbances, thyroid disorders, alcohol and other drugs, caffeine and smoking. Drugs are required only in hemodynamically unstable patients. Digoxin, metoprolol, diltiazem and quinidine may be used in pregnancy. Amiodarone is not safe. DC cardioversion is safe for the fetus.

In cases of prosthetic valves and AF, anticoagulation need consideration in pregnancy. Warfarin crosses placental and can cause a variety of fetal defects. The highest risk is form conception to 14th week and the risk increases with the dose. Heparin is dangerous to the mother and safer for baby. There are no clear-cut guidelines for anticoagulation in pregnancy. Some have advocated subcutaneous heparin before conception till delivery whereas some give warfarin in 2nd and 3rd trimester and switch back to heparin about 2 weeks before expected delivery date. But many patients may come after conception and continue warfarin with hardly any fetal effects. LMWH are inadequate as they cause thrombosis and embolism from prosthetic valves.

Endocarditis prophylaxis is advocated even for vaginal delivery for prosthetic valves, complex congenital defects, previous endocarditis and MVP. It is not required for ASD, or a previously repaired VSD or PDA.

Delivery: For most patients vaginal delivery is safer than cesarian section except in Marfan's syndrome. After delivery the placental blood is thrown in systemic circulation and may precipitate symptoms. The strapping of legs up in stirrups for delivery may also increase venous return to heart and cause problems. Cardiac output may remain up for several weeks after delivery especially if breastfeeding is going on.

Congenital Heart Disease

Left-to-right shunts: In the absence of significant symptoms or pulmonary hypertension, the outcome of pregnancy is usually normal and uncomplicated because the left-to-right shunting tends to diminish with the normal fall in systemic vascular resistance during pregnancy. Heart failure and arrhythmias are to be treated appropriately.

Right-to-left shunts: Eisenmenger's syndrome occurs as a result of right-to-left shunting through an intracardiac shunt due to development of fixed and high pulmonary vascular resistance. It is associated with a 30–50 percent maternal mortality during pregnancy. The decline in systemic vascular resistance that occurs during pregnancy results in an increase in right-to-left shunting and marked oxygen desaturation of blood. Pregnancy is contraindicated and sterilization should be recommended. If abortion is not feasible or the patient wants to continue with the pregnancy, supportive measures in the form of prevention of hypotension, hypovolemia and thromboembolism should be undertaken. Management strategies should include early hospitalization, anticoagulant therapy during the last 8–10 weeks of gestation and for 4 weeks postpartum, high concentrations of inhaled oxygen during noninduced vaginal delivery and attempts to shorten the second stage of labor by use of forceps.

Peripartum Cardiomyopathy

This is a dilated cardiomyopathy that can occur in the last month of pregnancy or upto 6 months after delivery in women without prior heart disease or reason to develop heart failure. It is estimated to occur with a frequency of 1 in 1300 to 1 in 4000 deliveries. PPCM occurs more frequently in older mothers, in term pregnancies, with toxemia and with multiparity. The peak incidence is at 1–2 months postpartum.

Etiology: The cause is not known. The interaction of viral and immune factors may play a role in producing myocardial injury. It is seen more in blacks, maternal age more than 30, multiparity, twin pregnancy, malnutrition, hypertension or toxemia of pregnancy. It recurs in 50 percent of subsequent pregnancies even if left ventricular function has retuned to normal in between. A second episode is worse than the first and probably fatal. This is an indication for preventing future pregnancy.

Treatment: This is as for any heart failure with the exception of avoiding ACE inhibitors and ARBs which can affect the fetal kidneys and should be avoided. Hydralazine and/or calcium channel blockers should be used to reduce afterload.

Prognosis: More than half of the patients recover. The prognosis is good if LVEF and LV size return to normal in 6 months. If there are symptoms late after delivery, severe LV dysfunction, marked LV enlargement or new LBBB the prognosis is worse. Mortality associated with PPCM is high, ranging from 25–50 percent, the majority of deaths occurring in the first year after delivery.

Systemic Hypertension During Pregnancy

This can be due to preexisting hypertension or it may develop de novo and is due to pregnancy itself (Pregnancy induced Hypertension).

Specific risks to the fetus include intrauterine growth retardation or death, placental insufficiency and premature delivery. Risks to the mother include left ventricular failure, cerebral hemorrhage and predisposition to toxemia. A raised blood pressure observed before the 20th week of gestation should be regarded as unrelated to pregnancy. If general measures such as adequate rest and salt restriction fail to control the blood pressure consistently below 150/90 mmHg the introduction of antihypertensive drug therapy is desirable. methyldopa, labetolol and hydralazine have been safely used for treating hypertension during pregnancy. Nifedipine sublingually may be used to tide over the crisis till the above drugs start acting. ACE inhibitors and ARBs are contraindicated.

Management of hypertensive crisis during pregnancy: Pregnancy with hypertensive crisis with or without superadded pre-eclampsia or the diastolic blood pressure rising abruptly by more than 40 mmHg requires urgent therapy to save the mother from pulmonary edema or from cerebral or retinal hemorrhage.

Drugs needed during this period are:

1. Hydralazine injected IV or IM in a dose of 10–20 mg followed by 100 mg added to a saline drip. The total daily dose should not exceed 400 mg.

2. Labetolol 20–80 mg given IV over 10 minutes.

3. Methyldopa 500–1000 mg IV 4–8 hourly.

4. Diazoxide in a rapid IV dose of 300 mg. It should preferably be avoided as there is increased fetal mortality.

5. Nitroprusside infusion at the rate of 0.03–0.5 mg/min. It should preferably be avoided. Diazoxide and nitroprusside are unsafe drugs but in emergency situations these may be used if other measures fail.

Pericardial Disease

The normal pericardium has two layers, the inner visceral and the outer parietal. In between the two layers is a small amount of pericardial fluid, usually less than 50 mL. This fluid is thought to originate from the visceral pericardium and is essentially an ultrafiltrate of plasma. Only the lower one-third of the parietal pericardium is sensitive to pain.

Pericarditis

Inflammation of the pericardium may be either acute or chronic.
1. *Acute*: This may be dry or effusive.
2. *Chronic*: It is generally constrictive but may also be effusive.

Etiology

There are various causes of acute pericarditis:
a. Idiopathic or nonspecific pericarditis
b. Rheumatic pericarditis
c. Infective
   – Viral (coxsackievirus A and B, and hepatitis viruses)
   – Bacterial: Tuberculosis, pyogenic organisms
   – Fungal
   – Parasitic: Echinococcus, amebiasis and filariasis
   – HIV
d. Metabolic disease, e.g. uremia
e. Collagen disorders, e.g. systemic lupus erythematosus
f. Postmyocardial infarction
g. Postoperative (common after cardiac surgery)
h. Neoplasms of the pericardium (primary or secondary)
i. Trauma
j. Endocrine disorders, e.g. myxedema
k. Drugs, e.g. hydralazine
l. Others like serum sickness, radiation.

Pathology

Acute pericarditis may be either dry or with effusion. Dry pericarditis is also called "bread and butter" pericarditis, as it gives such an appearance when the two layers are separated. Pericarditis with effusion results in the presence of fluid between the two layers of the pericardium. The fluid may be an exudate, or may contain blood (hemopericardium), pus (pyopericardium) or chyle (chylopericardium).

The pericardial reaction may be part of a generalized disorder (as in rheumatic fever and collagen disease) or may be due to a local cause (e.g. infection or trauma). The infection in pericarditis may be blood-borne, or a spread from neighboring structures (infection by contiguity) or introduced from outside (e.g. stab wounds).

Dry Pericarditis

Synonym: Acute fibrinous pericarditis

Clinical Features

Dry pericarditis may present with local or generalized symptoms. General symptoms include fever, bodyache, malaise, joint pains, anorexia.

Specific symptoms include chest pain and difficulty in breathing. The chest pain is localized to the sternal or parasternal area, but may occur allover the precordium. It is of a sharp stabbing nature which may be aggravated with inspiration, coughing and sneezing. It may be referred to the left shoulder, scapula and epigastrium. The pain is aggravated in the supine position and relieved by sitting up.

Though dyspnea is more common in pericarditis with effusion, it may also occur in dry pericarditis.

Signs

The patient may appear toxic and uncomfortable. A pericardial friction rub may be palpable over the precordium. The characteristic sign is the "pericardial rub" heard on auscultation. It is superficial, grating and has been described as resembling the creaking of leather. It has a to-and-fro character, is heard both in systole and in diastole, and is best audible in the third, fourth and fifth left intercostal spaces near the sternal edge, though the location may change with the position of the patient. It is better heard when the patient sits up and leans forward, and is heard louder if the stethoscope is pressed against the chest wall. Sometimes only the systolic or the diastolic component may be heard, and the rub may be mistaken for a murmur.

Besides the cardiac findings, other findings on general examination like joint swelling and rashes may be found.

Diagnosis

The characteristic pericardial rub is diagnostic. ECG shows ST elevation with concavity upwards. Changes in blood count, erythrocyte sedimentation rate, blood chemistry and other laboratory evidence identify and are specific for the underlying disease process.

Prognosis

This is dependent on the cause. Acute benign or idiopathic pericarditis has an excellent prognosis, while the pericarditis of uremia is usually a terminal event. Pericarditis due to rheumatic fever has a good prognosis. Few cases of viral pericarditis progress to constrictive pericarditis.

Treatment

The primary aim is to treat the cause of pericarditis. Thus anti-tubercular and antirheumatic treatment should be instituted whenever required. Supportive therapy like salicylates and corticosteroids provide symptomatic relief and may prevent adhesions. Appropriate antibiotic therapy is required for purulent pericarditis. Fever and pain need analgesic treatment.

Pericarditis with Effusion

Synonym: Exudative pericarditis

It may start as dry pericarditis with late development of effusion. In India, tuberculosis is the commonest cause. The quantity of pericardial fluid may vary from 150–1000 mL or more. The fluid is an exudate and may contain pus, blood or chyle.

Clinical Features
Symptoms
They are essentially the same as those of dry pericarditis, but the dyspnea may be more marked. Dyspnea is considered to be secondary to compression of the lungs and bronchi, and encroachment on the intrathoracic space. The dyspnea is characteristically relieved in the sitting up and leaning forward position (Mohammedan prayer position) probably because in this position the fluid gravitates forward and downwards, exerting less pressure on the lungs and bronchi.

If the effusion is large and produces sufficient pressure on the bronchi, it may result in a dry hacking cough, hoarseness of voice, and difficulty in swallowing.

Signs
A cyanotic tinge may be observed occasionally. A paradoxical arterial pulse with diminution of the volume in inspiration is characteristic. This may be further corroborated by the use of sphygmomanometer. A reduction of systolic blood pressure by 10 mmHg or more during inspiration is diagnostic. This is a misnomer and is actually an exaggeration of normal fall of blood pressure during inspiration. The neck veins are full and even fuller during deep inspiration (Kussmaul's sign). There may be edema on the legs, ascites and a palpable tender liver.

Examination of the heart reveals the apex beat to be either weakly palpable or it may not be palpable at all. Bulging of the precordium and xiphisternum may be seen. However in some patients the apex beat continues to be well palpable. A pericardial friction rub may occasionally be palpated.

Percussion of the heart reveals an increase in the area of cardiac dullness especially on the left side. The dullness over the left second space decreases (shifting dullness) when the patient sits up and the fluid gravitates downwards. There is an area of dullness on the right side of the sternum in the fifth intercostal space (Rotch's sign). Percussion of the back reveals an area of dullness in the left infrascapular region, with bronchial breathing and aegophony (Ewart's sign) due to compression of the base of the left lung. Characteristically, if the apex beat is palpable, the area of dullness extends significantly beyond the apex.

On auscultation, the heart sounds are very soft (muffled). However, occasionally, they are normally heard. A pericardial rub may be occasionally heard, though it tends to disappear with accumulation of fluid. Marked fluid accumulation leads to cardiac tamponade.

Cardiac Tamponade

Definition

It has been described as "impaired diastolic filling of the ventricles due to rising intrapericardial pressure".

Hemodynamics

The impaired diastolic filling is associated with decrease in stroke volume. Though cardiac tamponade is due to an increase in pericardial fluid, it is observed more commonly when the amount of fluid increases rapidly. Large pericardial effusion which accumulates gradually may not result in tamponade.

Due to the high intrapericardial pressure, ventricular filling is restricted and the ventricular diastole is restricted with associated rise of pressure. The stroke output and the minute output decrease as the rising intrapericardial pressure interferes with venous inflow and compensatory tachycardia becomes ineffective. Eventually the systemic pressure also decreases.

Clinical Features

Cardiac tamponade is suspected in a patient who has a rapid downhill course and exhibits classic Beck triad of pericardial tamponade of (1) rising systemic venous pressure, (2) falling arterial pressure and (3) a quiet heart (muffled heart sounds). Along with this, tachycardia is also observed. The patient usually sits up and leans forward or may assume a knee-chest position. Other signs of pericardial effusion are also present. The patient is generally restless, anxious and cyanotic or pale.

Untreated cardiac tamponade is generally fatal; it requires urgent pericardial aspiration.

Investigations

There may be leukocytosis and neutrophilia, and the erythrocyte sedimentation rate may be high. Other investigations include determination of ASO titers, C-reactive proteins, and specific investigations for the underlying etiological cause including viral studies and TSH.

Electrocardiogram: The electrocardiographic changes are quite characteristic. Initially the ST segment is elevated in all leads with concavity upwards with PR depression. This is in contrast to myocardial infarction where the elevation has the convexity upwards. Unlike myocardial infarction there is no reciprocal depression of the ST segment in pericarditis. The T waves are upright to begin with but become flat and later inverted along with the return of the ST segment to the isoelectric position. These changes may persist for as long as six months or more.

Associated with these changes sinus tachycardia and diminution in QRS voltage are commonly present.

Chest X-ray: In dry pericarditis, fluoroscopy reveals no abnormality. In patients with pericardial effusion, the cardiac silhouette is variably increased in size. This may be more noticeable in serial roentgenograms. The individual chamber and blood vessel contours are lost. Cardiac pulsations are markedly reduced. If the patient is examined in the Trendelenburg position, the cardiac silhouette changes its shape as the fluid gravitates downwards (Fig. 10.1).

It is one of the most useful investigations to document pericardial effusion which is seen as an echo-free space behind the left ventricular posterior echoes (depicted by arrow in Fig. 10.2). In larger effusion fluid may be present anteriorly. Pericardial effusions are described as small, moderate, or large based on the size of the echo-free space seen between the parietal and visceral pleurae on 2-dimensional echocardiography. Small effusions have an echo-free space of less than 5 mm, and are generally seen posteriorly. Moderate-sized effusions range from 5–10 mm

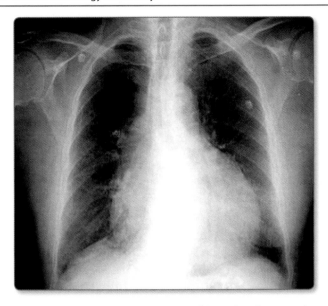

Fig. 10.1: Note the "water-bottle" appearance of the cardiac silhouette in the anteroposterior (AP) chest film

and are circumferential, and greater than 10 mm indicates a large effusion. Fluid adjacent to the right atrium is an early sign of pericardial effusion. In case of gross effusion, the apical four-chamber view reveals the heart to move rapidly from side to side, the so-called "swinging heart".

Cardiac catheterization: The introduction of a cardiac catheter into the right atrium, abutting against the lateral atrial wall, will denote the quantity of pericardial fluid.

Diagnostic pericardiocentesis: Aspiration of the pericardial fluid will not only confirm the diagnosis but may also help identify the underlying etiology. The aspirated fluid should be sent for microscopic, chemical, microbiological and other required tests. Other investigative methods include pericardial biopsy and radioisotope scanning.

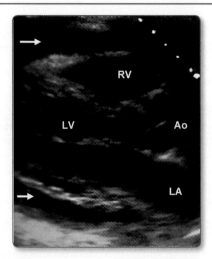

Fig. 10.2: Echocardiography showing pericardial effusion (arrow)

Differential Diagnosis

Pericardial effusion has to be differentiated from other causes of cardiomegaly such as cardiomyopathy, cardiac failure and Ebstein's anomaly of the tricuspid valve. The change in cardiac silhouette in the Trendelenburg position, the characteristic electrocardiographic abnormalities, a paradoxical pulse and the presence of a pericardial friction rub are useful in arriving at the diagnosis.

Prognosis

This depends on the etiological factor. Tuberculous pericarditis frequently results in chronic constrictive pericarditis. Idiopathic pericarditis and rheumatic pericarditis have a good prognosis and heal without any sequelae. Purulent pericarditis, if not treated vigorously, may prove fatal; even when adequately treated it may lead to rapid development of constrictive pericarditis.

Treatment

The treatment of pericardial effusion is two-fold:
1. Treatment of the etiological factor
2. Treatment of the effusion.

Pericardiocentesis

The indications for therapeutic paracentesis are cardiac tamponade, relief of dyspnea and the introduction of cytotoxic drugs into the pericardial cavity. Air may be injected into the pericardial cavity after the fluid is aspirated to determine the underlying cardiac size and for assessment of the thickness of the pericardium.

Procedure: The patient is premedicated with a sedative and atropine. The skin over the precordium and upper abdomen is prepared as for a surgical procedure. Under local anesthesia, a needle connected to a syringe via a two-way stop-cock is introduced into the pericardial cavity, and the fluid is aspirated. Depending on the quantity various sites are used for aspiration. The two common sites are the epigastric region and the left fifth intercostal space. The epigastric site is generally preferred since small effusions can be aspirated. The aspiration needle is introduced between the xiphisternum and the left costal arch and is directed superiorly and to the left at an angle of 45°. As soon as it enters the pericardial cavity the fluid can be aspirated. During the procedure if frank blood is withdrawn, then the tip of the needle is drawn and repositioned. Aspiration should preferably be done under image intensifier control and with all resuscitative facilities available.

If the fluid withdrawn is found to be purulent, the pericardial cavity should be drained with an indwelling tube connected to an under-water seal. Along with this, appropriate antibiotic therapy should be given. Pericardial sclerosis for malignant effusion:
- Several pericardial sclerosing agents have been used with varying success rates (e.g. tetracycline, doxycycline, cisplatin, and 5-fluorouracil).

- The pericardial catheter may be left in place for repeat instillation if necessary until the effusion resolves.
- Complications include intense pain, atrial dysrhythmias, fever, and infection.
- Success rates are reported as high as 91 percent at 30 days.

Rheumatic Pericarditis

This is seen as part of acute rheumatic fever with carditis and is characterized by tachycardia, chest pain and fleeting joint pains or arthritis. The pericarditis is usually dry but occasionally significant effusion may develop. The pericarditis regresses completely with treatment and subsequent chronic pericarditis does not occur.

Tuberculosis Pericarditis

This is the commonest cause of pericarditis in India. Infection of the pericardium occurs by spread from neighboring structures, e.g. lungs, bronchi, lymph nodes, or is blood-borne. Often, even a close search may reveal no evidence of tuberculosis anywhere else in the body.

The patient may have vague complaints like fever, malaise, evening rise in temperature and loss of weight. The cardiac manifestations may be absent to begin with. Later on, chest pain, cough and dyspnea may appear, due to an increase in the size of pericardial effusion. This may progress to the development of ascites and edema of the feet.

Aspiration reveals either a straw-colored or hemorrhagic fluid, which is an exudate with predominant lymphocytes. Culture may reveal the presence of tubercle bacilli.

The initial treatment of tuberculous pericarditis should include isoniazid 300 mg/day, rifampin 450–600 mg/day, pyrazinamide 15–30 mg/kg/day, and ethambutol 15–25 mg/kg/day. Prednisone 1–2 mg/kg/day is given for 5–7 days and progressively reduced to discontinuation in 6–8 weeks. Uncertainty remains whether adjunctive corticosteroids are effective in reducing mortality or progression to constriction. Surgical resection of the pericardium remains the appropriate treatment for constrictive pericarditis. The timing of surgical intervention is controversial, but many experts recommend a trial of medical therapy for noncalcific pericardial constriction and pericardiectomy in nonresponders after 4–8 weeks of antituberculosis chemotherapy.

Purulent Pericarditis

This is commonly caused by infection of the pericardium by organisms like staphylococci, streptococci, pneumococci, meningococci and *Hemophilus influenzae*. The infection may be blood-borne, may extend from an intrathoracic infection or may be introduced from outside as in stab wounds.

The clinical features of pericarditis may be obscured by those of the primary disease. The patient has high fever and is very toxic in appearance. If the effusion accumulates rapidly, features of cardiac tamponade result. The presence of a pericardial rub is diagnostic. Chronic constrictive pericarditis may result early or late in the course of purulent pericarditis.

Treatment consists of drainage of the pericardium and appropriate antibiotic therapy instituted early. Pericardiectomy has also been recommended in the acute stages. This is especially so when the patient fails to respond to antibiotic therapy and to drainage.

Chronic Constrictive Pericarditis

Definition

Chronic constrictive pericarditis is defined as a dense and rigid thickening of one or both layers of the pericardium with adhesions, resulting in compression of the heart with impairment in diastolic filling.

Etiology

In India, a majority (50%) of cases are the end-result of tuberculous pericarditis. In some cases the disease is bacterial or neoplastic in origin. However, in a significant number of patients, the etiology may not be determinable. The disease occurs at all ages, commonly in the young.

Pathology

The pericardium is thickened and may be calcified (the normal thickness of the pericardium is 3–5 mm). The thickened pericardium forms an encasement over the heart which is unable to stretch during diastole. As a result, the heart may appear to be smaller than normal. The liver is enlarged and its capsule is thickened. The spleen may be enlarged as a consequence of chronic congestion.

Clinical Features

The commonest complaint is that of distension of the abdomen due to ascites. Dyspnea, swelling of the feet, fatigue and loss of weight are also frequent. Loss of weight is common if allowance is made for serous effusions and oedema.

On inspection, the veins are markedly engorged even in the erect position. A deep 'Y' descent (Freidrich's sign) is seen. An increase in the fullness of the veins on deep inspiration (Kussmaul's sign) is common.

The arterial pulse is of low volume and pulsus parodoxus is frequently present. The rhythm may be irregular indicating the presence of atrial fibrillation (5%). There may be pitting edema on the feet. Occasionally a cyanotic tinge may be observed.

Inspection of the precordium reveals a 'quiet' heart and prominent veins may be seen all over the chest wall. A systolic retraction at the apex may be observed. A systolic 'tap' or 'shock' due to rapid filling of the right ventricle during early diastole may be palpable.

The characteristic finding on auscultation is the 'pericardial knock'. This is a sound due to rapid filling of the ventricle in the early rapid filling phase. It occurs about 0.08–0.12 second after the second sound in contrast to the normal third sound which occurs a little later (0.13–0.16 second). The heart sounds are normal and murmurs are prominent by their absence.

The liver is markedly enlarged, firm, smooth and tender. It is usually pulsatile. Hepatic and splenic enlargement occurs quite early in the course of the disease. Ascites is invariably present and is usually massive, and out of proportion to the edema on the legs which may be minimal. It tends to recur rapidly after aspiration (Table 10.1).

Investigations

Electrocardiogram: The electrocardiographic findings are not characteristic but include low voltage of the QRS complexes, flattening or inversion of T waves and occasionally atrial fibrillation.

Roentgenology: The heart size is usually normal or may be slightly smaller. Uncommonly, a slight cardiomegaly is seen. Cardiac pulsations are either diminished or absent. The superior vena caval shadow is prominent. The characteristic finding is calcification of the pericardium best seen in the left lateral or oblique views but is present in less than 50 percent of established cases (Fig. 10.3, depicted by arrow). The cardiac silhouette may have a shaggy appearance. Left atrial enlargement is present (30–40%). Lung fields are usually clear. Unilateral or bilateral pleural effusion may be present.

Echocardiography will show thickened and at times calcifies pericardium and features of collapse of cavities.

Diagnosis

The combination of pulsus paradoxus, venous engorgement with prominent 'Y' descent, ascites and pericardial 'knock' eases the diagnosis of constrictive pericarditis. However, a similar

Table 10.1: Salient features of constrictive pericarditis

1. Fast, low volume pulse
2. Pulsus paradoxsus (BP falls > 10 mmHg during inspiration)
3. Raised JVP with rapid Y descent
4. JVP increases during inspiration (paradoxical)—Kussmaul's sign
5. Pericardial knock on auscultation
6. Enlarged tender liver
7. Ascites and dependent edema of feet

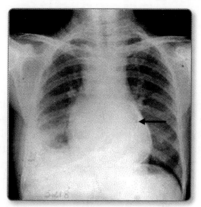

Fig. 10.3: Chest X-ray showing pericardial calcification

clinical picture may be present in tricuspid valvular disease, cardiomyopathy and cirrhosis of the liver. Tricuspid valvular diseases, however, have their characteristic cardiac murmurs on auscultation. Cardiomyopathy may pose difficulties and may sometimes be indistinguishable even at cardiac catheterization. Cirrhosis of the liver can be distinguished from constrictive pericarditis by the absence of systemic venous hypertension.

Prognosis

Without surgery the prognosis is poor. Long-standing cases develop hypoproteinemia due to protein-losing enteropathy. They also develop myocardial dysfunction (presumably due to fibrosis) which does not respond to digoxin, even after pericardiectomy.

Treatment

The treatment is surgical and consists of pericardial resection. However, in patients with suspected tuberculous pericarditis a few weeks of antituberculous treatment should precede surgery. The results of surgery are generally gratifying.

Endocarditis

Lazare Riviere first described gross autopsy findings of the disease in 1723. In 1885, William Osler presented the first comprehensive description of endocarditis in English. Lerner and Weinstein presented a thorough discussion of this disease in modern times in their landmark series of articles, "Infective Endocarditis in the Antibiotic Era," published in 1966 in the New England Journal of Medicine.

Definition: Infective endocarditis (IE) is defined as microbial infection of the endocardium. The characteristic lesion is vegetation commonly seen on diseased heart valves or a congenital defect. IE may be either acute or subacute depending upon the rapidity of the development of the disease and the virulence of the organism. Rapidly progressive disease over a few days, commonly due to *Staphylococcus aureus,* is termed acute infective endocarditis whereas IE developing over a period of a few weeks due to organisms of low virulence like *Streptococcus viridans* is called subacute bacterial endocarditis (SBE).

Infection could develop in prosthetic heart valves, prosthetic valve endocarditis (PVE), and rarely vegetations are seen in some chronic diseases and malignancy (nonbacterial thrombotic endocarditis). Eventually, 5 percent of mechanical and bioprosthetic valves become infected. Mechanical valves are more likely to be infected within the first 3 months of implantation, and after 1 year, bioprosthetic valves are more likely to be infected. The valves in the mitral valve position are more susceptible than those in the aortic areas.

Analogous to PVE are infections of implantable pacemakers and cardioverter-defibrillators. Usually, these devices are infected within a few months of implantation. Infection of pacemakers includes that of the generator pocket (the most common), infection of the proximal leads, and infection of the portions of the leads in direct contact with the endocardium. This last category represents true pacemaker IE, is the least common infectious complication of pacemakers (0.5% of implanted pacemakers), and is the most challenging to treat. Of pacemaker infections, 75 percent are produced by staphylococci, both coagulase-negative and coagulase-positive.

Incidence

In the US the incidence of IE is approximately 2–4 cases per 100,000 persons per year.

Changing Pattern

Since the availability of antibiotics, the disease pattern has changed considerably, as follows:

- Mean age of patients has increased from 30–50 years
- Male to female ratio has increased
- Incidence of infection due to *Staphylococcus aureus* and fungi has increased significantly especially among intravenous drug abusers (IVDA)
- Incidence of IE without preexisting cardiac disease has also increased
- The so-called 'classical' signs of SBE like Osler nodes, Janeway lesions, clubbing, and Roth spots are seen much less frequently
- The incidence of IE has increased among operated cardiac cases [prosthetic valve endocarditis (PVE), corrected congenital defects] probably due to increased longevity of patients
- IE may occur with mitral valve prolapse
- Right heart endocarditis is being noted more often, especially in intravenous drug abusers
- Nosocomial infective endocarditis (NIE) has markedly increased. Valvular infections have entered the era of IE caused by intravascular devices and procedures.

Pathogenesis and Pathology

Host factors: The middle-aged and elderly are more prone to IE; in contrast, the disease is uncommon in children less than 2 years of age. It is much more common in males (M:F 4:1) especially because of the increasing incidence of intravenous drug abuse. SBE generally occurs in diseased heart valves or congenital defect (Table 11.1). Rheumatic heart disease currently accounts for majority of cases. Approximately 50 percent of elderly patients have calcific aortic stenosis as the underlying pathology. Congenital heart disease accounts for 15 percent of cases, with the bicuspid aortic valve being the most common example. Other contributing congenital abnormalities include ventricular septal defects, patent ductus arteriosus, and tetralogy of Fallot. Atrial septal defect (secundum variety) is rarely associated with IE. Mitral valve prolapse is the most common predisposing condition found in young adults and is the predisposing condition in 30 percent of cases of native valve endocarditis (NVE) in this age group.

IE is distinctly uncommon in atherosclerotic coronary artery disease, hypertension and syphilitic heart disease.

Table 11.1: Risk of infective endocarditis in various cardiac lesions

High-risk	Moderate risk	Low-risk
Prosthetic heart valves (aortic, mitral)	Mitral valve prolapse with mitral regurgitation	Mitral valve prolapse without mitral regurgitation
Tetralogy of Fallot especially with BT shunt	Tricuspid stenosis	
Patent ductus arteriosus	Tricuspid regurgitation	
Aortic regurgitation	Pulmonic stenosis	Atrial septal defect
Aortic stenosis	Mitral stenosis	
Coarctation of aorta		
Ventricular septal defect		
Mitral regurgitation		

Microbes: SBE is commonly caused by organisms of low virulence like *Streptococcus viridans, Streptococcus bovis, Streptococcus faecalis,* and *Staphylococcus epidermidis.* Rarely it could also be caused by gram-negative organisms, diphtheroids, fungi or other organisms. *Staphylococcus aureus* is becoming a major cause especially in developed countries and more than half are due to underlying valve disease. *S. aureus* IE carries a high mortality of 40–50 percent. *S. viridans* causes 50–60 percent subacute IE. Approximately 5 percent of cases of possible IE yield negative blood culture results (i.e. culture-negative IE). These may have noninfectious causes (e.g. vasculitis) or may be caused by fastidious organisms (Fig. 11.1).

The diagnostic pathologic lesion of SBE is the development of a vegetation which is either sessile or a polypoidal mobile mass situated on the heart leaflets defects. A vegetation is formed when platelets and fibrin get deposited on the diseased valves forming small masses. The microbes then gain access to these sterile fibrin platelet masses producing localized inflammation and more platelet and fibrin deposition occurs enmeshing the microbes, resulting into growth of the vegetation.

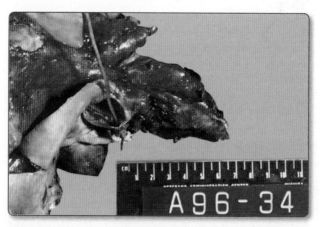

Fig. 11.1: Acute bacterial endocarditis caused by *Staphylococcus aureus* with perforation of the aortic valve (shown by a probe) and aortic valve vegetations

Commonly, the bacteria gain entry into the circulation by way of an untreated or partially treated septic focus (abscess, pneumonia, urinary tract infection) or by diagnostic or therapeutic instrumentation (different types of endoscopies, operative procedures, dental surgery) or along indwelling venous and arterial cannulae or intravenous catheters used for long-term feeding.

The vegetations may embolize to the central nervous system leading to hemiplegia, meningitis, intracerebral hemorrhage, encephalopathy and, at a later date, rupture of mycotic aneurysms resulting in hemorrhage; or the abdomen (i.e. liver, spleen, kidneys, intestines); or to the extremities resulting in digital gangrene. In the case of right heart endocarditis, embolized vegetations lodge in the lungs, leading to pneumonia, lung abscess and empyema.

Untreated, SBE commonly leads to heart failure either due to a mechanical complication of the cardiac valve (rupture/ perforation) or due to an inflammatory myocarditis. Besides embolic phenomena and heart failure, SBE is also known to evoke an intense immune response which may sometimes manifest clinically in the form of pericarditis, arthritis and renal failure.

IE develops most commonly on the mitral valve, closely followed in descending order of frequency by the aortic valve, the combined mitral and aortic valve, the tricuspid valve, and, rarely, the pulmonic valve. Mechanical prosthetic and bioprosthetic valves exhibit equal rates of infection.

Clinical Features

The diagnosis of IE requires a high degree of suspicion in any patient with a murmur and unexplained fever. The classic clinical presentation and clinical course of IE has been characterized as either acute or subacute. Acute IE frequently involves normal valves. It is a rapidly progressive illness in persons who are healthy or debilitated. Subacute IE typically affects only abnormal valves. Its course, even in untreated patients, may extend over many months.

Subacute Infective Endocarditis

Symptoms: The diagnosis of subacute infective endocarditis (IE) is suggested by a history of an indolent process characterized by fever, fatigue, anorexia, back pain, and weight loss. Less common developments include a cerebrovascular accident or congestive heart failure.

Signs: The cardinal features on examination (Fig. 11.2) are pyrexia, pallor, petechiae, palpable spleen and clubbing of digits. Fever is always present and is usually moderate to high. Clubbing of fingers and toes was found almost universally, but it is now observed in less often. It primarily occurs in those patients who have an extended course of untreated IE. Splenomegaly is observed more commonly in patients with long-standing subacute disease. It may persist long after successful therapy. Cardiac examination reveals murmurs pertaining to the underlying heart disease and one may find change in character of murmurs due to development of endocarditis. According to some authorities the saying "a changing murmur is extremely

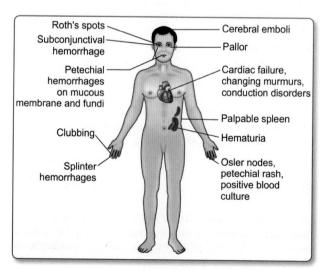

Fig. 11.2: Clinical features of infective endocarditis

helpful in diagnosing subacute IE" is a myth. Only 15 percent do so early in the course of infection.

Signs of heart failure may develop. The spleen is small and soft and nontender except when there is infarct or abscess. Apart from the skin, petechiae may be seen in the oral cavity, conjunctivae and even on the retina. Petechiae are probably due to microembolization of small vessels.

The other features of IE listed below are seen much less frequently probably due to early diagnosis.

Splinter hemorrhages are linear, subungual, dark red streaks especially in the fingers, less commonly in the toes. They are probably due to embolism to the linear capillaries in the nail bed.

Osler's nodes are painful, tender, pea-sized erythematous nodules in the pulp of fingers which tend to occur in crops and are indicator either of embolism to distal digital arteries or an immunological phenomenon.

Janeway's lesions are small (< 5 mm), maculopapular, erythematous or hemorrhagic, nontender lesions commonly seen on the thenar and hypothenar eminences of the hands and feet, blanching on pressure. They are thought to be of embolic origin.

Eye lesions: Apart from petechial hemorrhages retinal hemorrhages which are rounded or flame-shaped with a central clearing and due to embolization are occasionally seen. (Roth spots). The Litten sign represents cotton-wool exudates. There may be sudden loss of vision in one eye secondary to embolization of a large retinal artery.

Complications

Heart failure: Endocarditis may precipitate or aggravate heart failure and this is the single most important complication responsible for high morbidity and mortality. Heart failure may occur following a tear in a leaflet, ruptured chordae tendinae, dehiscence of a prosthetic valve or perforation of the interventricular septum. Alternatively, heart failure may be secondary to inflammatory myocarditis.

Embolization can occur to any organ in the body.

Renal failure: Fortunately, due to early diagnosis, the frequency of this complication has become much less.

Diagnosis

Investigations done for diagnosis of endocarditis are shown in Table 11.2.

Differential Diagnosis

Subacute bacterial endocarditis (SBE) should be considered an important differential diagnosis in any patient with unexplained

Table 11.2: Investigations for diagnosis of endocarditis

1. Anemia is almost universal and is normochromic, normocytic
2. Leukocyte count is generally normal or mildly elevated
3. Platelet counts are generally normal, rarely low
4. Erythrocyte sedimentation rate: A moderate to high sedimentation rate is almost universal
5. Urine examination reveals mild albuminuria and microscopic hematuria
6. In long-standing untreated cases, there may be immune activation resulting in positive RA factor and VDRL test
7. Echocardiogram: Vegetations may be identified as small, sessile or polypoidal masses on heart valves or congenital defects (Fig. 11.3). Transesophageal echocardiogram, which has greater than 90–95 percent accuracy, may be used. However, failure to detect vegetations on echocardiogram does not rule out endocarditis. Besides vegetations, echocardiography also provides useful information about the underlying cardiac lesion, ventricular function and complications like perforation of leaflets, chordal rupture and septal perforation
8. Blood culture: The sine qua non of infective endocarditis is the recovery of the microorganisms causing the IE from the circulation. Generally, 4–6 samples are withdrawn for culture before administering antibiotics over 24 hours. Blood cultures collected just prior to the expected temperature peak give a higher yield
9. Electrocardiography may help detect the 10 percent of patients who develop a conduction delay during IE by documenting an increased P-R interval

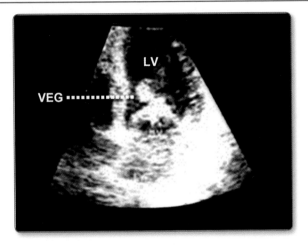

Fig. 11.3: Echocardiogram showing vegetations on the mitral valve

fever with a heart murmur. The differential diagnosis includes tuberculosis, malaria, osteomyelitis, glomerulonephritis, recurrent pneumonias (especially for right heart endocarditis), rheumatic fever, enteric fever and connective tissue disorders.

Treatment

Untreated SBE carries a high morbidity and is generally fatal. The microbes in the vegetations are partly protected from the action of antibiotics, being deep-seated and surrounded by a fibrin mesh in the relatively poorly vascularized vegetation masses. Hence, only bactericidal antibiotics in large doses should be administered frequently by the parenteral route for a period of 4 to 6 weeks, with the hope of destroying the microbes completely and preventing recurrence of infection. The commonly used drug regimes are given in Table 11.3.

In addition to antibiotic therapy, the patient must be given complete bed rest, properly regulated fluids, electrolytes and diet and the other medications as dictated by an individual case like digoxin, diuretics and ACE inhibitors for heart failure; whole blood or packed cell transfusions for severe anemia; and hematinics for milder anemia when due to iron or folic acid deficiency.

Table 11.3: Antibiotics in infective endocarditis

Organism	Regimen
Streptococcus viridans	Penicillin G IV 4 million units 6 hourly for 4 weeks plus Gentamicin 1 mg/kg 8 hourly for 2 weeks
Streptococcus bovis	Gentamicin IV as above Ceftriaxone IV 2.0 g once daily (for penicillin allergic patients) Vancomycin IV 30 mg/kg/day in 2 divided doses (max 2.0 g/day) (for penicillin and cephalosporin allergic patients)
Enterococcus faecalis and other penicillin resistant streptococci	Ampicillin IV 2 g 4 hourly Gentamicin IV 1 mg/kg (max 80 mg) 8 hourly or (for penicillin allergic) Vancomycin, IV 30 mg/kg/day in 2 divided doses Gentamicin IV 1 mg/kg 8 hourly
Staphylococcus aureus	Nafcillin IV 2 g 4 hourly (additional gentamicin IV 1 mg/kg 8 hourly may be given for the first 3–5 days) Or (for penicillin allergic) Cefazolin IV 2 g 8 hourly. Additional gentamicin, IV 1 mg/kg 8 hourly may be given for the first 3–5 days. or (for penicillin and cephalosporin allergic) Vancomycin IV 30 mg/kg/day in 2 divided doses.
HACEK organisms (*Haemophilus parainfluenzae, Haemophilus aphrophilus, Actinobacillus (actinomycetemcomitans), Cardiobacterium hominis,* Eikenella corrodens, Kingella-kingae)	Ampicillin IV 2 g 4 hourly + Gentamicin 1 mg/kg 8 hourly or (for penicillin allergic) Ceftriaxone 2 g OD IV/IM
Enterobacteriaceae	Cefotaxime IV 8 g/day in 4 divided doses or Imipenem IV 2–4 g/day in 4 divided doses or Aztreonam IV 8 g/day in 4 divided doses Gentamicin 5 mg/kg/day in 3 divided doses
Pseudomonas aeruginosa	Piperacillin IV 18 g/day in 6 divided doses or Ceftazidime 6 g/day in 3 divided doses or Imipenem IV 2–4 g/day in 4 divided doses + Tobramycin IV 5 mg/kg/day in 3 divided doses or Aztreonam IV 8 g/day in 4 divided doses + Gentamicin 5 mg/kg/day in 3 divided doses
Fungi	Amphotericin B IV 1 mg/kg/day Flucytosine PO 150 mg/kg/day in 4 divided doses
Empiric therapy	Ampicillin IV 2 g 4 hourly Gentamicin IV 1 mg/kg 8 hourly

Most cases show a good response to treatment and four weeks of treatment suffice even for highly virulent organisms like staphylococci. For organisms known to be relatively resistant, like enterococci, gram-negative microbes and fungi, it is better to extend the therapy to 6 weeks to achieve higher cure rates.

Mortality rates for treated SBE range from 16–27 percent. Factors associated with a higher mortality include

a. Age above 65 years
b. Underlying medical disorders
c. Development of congestive heart failure
d. Major embolic complications especially to the central nervous system.

Mortality rates also depend on the infecting microbes, being much lower with *Streptococcus viridans* and *bovis* (less than 10%) but significantly higher with *Staphylococcus aureus*, Gram-negative organisms or fungi where it may be close to 50 percent.

Relapse and Recurrence

Relapse is seen within the first 2 months of cessation of therapy and blood culture reveals the same organisms, showing that the vegetations were not adequately sterilized during the previous drug therapy. Reinfection can occur at any time and may be due to the same or a different organism.

Acute Infective Endocarditis

The incidence of this type of endocarditis is low but when it occurs, it carries a high morbidity and mortality. The infection is caused by microbes like *Staphylococcus pyogenes*. The history is generally of a shorter duration with the patient looking very toxic. Embolic phenomena are common. The patient may be hemodynamically unstable or in frank congestive heart failure secondary to destruction of valvular heart structures and may need immediate surgical intervention beside medical treatment.

Leukocyte count and ESR are usually elevated. Four to six blood cultures from different venous sites should be drawn within half an hour and an instant echocardiogram carried out to look for vegetations, basic underlying pathology, ventricular function, presence of any new regurgitation secondary to valve destruction and pericardial effusion.

The patient should be treated empirically with antibiotic combinations which include antistaphylococcal agents till culture reports are available. One such recommended regime is as follows:

- Ampicillin IV 2 g 4 hourly
+
Nafcillin IV 2 g 4 hourly
+
Gentamicin IV 1 mg/kg 8 hourly
Or
- Vancomycin IV 30 mg/kg/day in 2 divided doses (for penicillin allergic patients)
+
Gentamicin 1 mg/kg 8 hourly

The patient should be watched closely for evidence of destruction of heart valves leading to acute regurgitation or development of myo-cardial abscesses leading to ventricular septal defect or sudden change in atrioventricular conduction (sometimes seen in aortic valve en-docarditis), in which case the patient will need to undergo appropriate surgical correction or pacemaker implantation without delay.

Prosthetic Valve Endocarditis

Patients with prosthetic valves are at higher risk for the development of IE compared to those with diseased native valves. Two types of PVE are described:

1. Early PVE, which occurs within 60 days of the surgery
2. Late PVE, after 60 days of surgery.

Early PVE commonly shows *Staphylococcus epidermidis* on culture isolates or mixed infections; therapy should preferably always be culture-guided, more so because some of these organisms may be hospital-acquired and hence resistant to commonly used antibiotics. Early PVE commonly occurs around 3–6 weeks postsurgery and needs to be aggressively investigated and treated along the lines of acute bacterial endocarditis. A significant proportion of patients with early PVE will need to undergo repeat valve replacement in order to eradicate the microbes completely.

Late PVE resembles subacute bacterial endocarditis of native valves and hence should be investigated and managed similarly.

Right-sided Endocarditis

With the increase in intravenous drug abuse, the incidence of right heart endocarditis has increased markedly. It may also occur in immunocompromised hosts including diabetics, cirrhotics, those with alcoholic liver disease, or on chemotherapy or steroids, and those with burns. A common presentation may be recurrent pneumonias, empyemas and lung abscesses. Blood cultures are a must before initiation of therapy since the microbes can range from a single organism to a host of mixed flora. Also, in the event of staphylococcal or fungal infections, the vegetation masses may be very large and show a partial to no response to adequate doses of antibiotics. Hence, treatment may include not only antibiotics but early surgery as well (Table 11.4).

Prophylaxis

Since endocarditis is a disease associated with high morbidity and mortality, it is worthwhile giving antibiotic prophylaxis to patients with underlying valvular or congenital heart

Table 11.4: Indications for surgery in infective endocarditis

1. Acute resistant heart failure secondary to mechanical complications like ruptured chordae, valve perforations or perforations of interventricular septum
2. Prosthetic valve dysfunction
3. Myocardial abscess
4. Large vegetations (more than 10 mm) with recurrent emboli
5. Infections with organisms which respond poorly to medical treatment, like fungi
6. Repeated relapses

Table 11.5: Common cardiac conditions for which endocarditis prophylaxis is recommended

1. Prosthetic cardiac valves
2. Rheumatic and other acquired valvular dysfunctions
3. Most congenital cardiac malformations
4. Surgically constructed systemic-pulmonary shunts
5. Idiopathic hypertrophic subaortic stenosis
6. Previous history of bacterial endocarditis
7. Mitral valve prolapse with insufficiency

diseases undergoing dental or invasive diagnostic procedures (endoscopies, minor or major surgical procedures) since they are all associated with transient bacteremias which may result in endocarditis (Table 11.5). The standard prophylactic antibiotic regimens for IE are given in Table 11.6.

Table 11.6: Infective endocarditis prophylaxis

Procedure	Regimen
Prophylaxis for dental, oral and upper respiratory procedures	*Oral regimen*
	Amoxicillin PO 3 g orally, one hour prior to procedure and 1.5 g PO 6 hours after first dose Or (for penicillin allergic patients) i. Erythromycin PO 1 g 2 hours prior to procedure and 0.5 g 6 hours after first dose. Or ii. Clindamycin 300 mg 1 hour before procedure and 150 mg 6 hours later
Prophylaxis for genitourinary and gastrointestinal procedures	*Parenteral regimens*
	Ampicillin IV 2 g 30 minutes before procedure and 1 g 6 hours later or Clindamycin IV 300 mg 30 minutes before procedure and 150 mg 6 hours later Ampicillin IV 2 g + Gentamicin IV 1.5 mg/kg 30 minutes before procedure followed by one dose 8 hours later of amoxicillin PO 1.5 g or (for penicillin allergic patients) Vancomycin IV 1 g + Gentamicin IV 1.5 mg/kg 1 hour prior to procedure, both to be repeated after 8 hours

We will include pulmonary hypertension, cor pulmonale and pulmonary embolism in this chapter.

Pulmonary Hypertension

Definition

Pulmonary artery pressure in an individual living at sea-level is 18–25/6–10 mmHg. Pulmonary hypertension (PH) exists when pulmonary artery systolic and mean pressure exceed 30 and 20 mmHg, respectively. The normal pulmonary vascular bed offers less than one-tenth the resistance to flow offered by the systemic bed. In normal adults, the pulmonary vascular resistance (PVR) is 67 ± 23 dynes-sec-cm-5 or roughly one Wood unit. PH results when PVR is increased (passive, obliterative, obstructive or vasoconstrictive PH) or when pulmonary blood flow is markedly increased (hyperkinetic PH). Common causes of PH are cardiac and respiratory diseases and pulmonary thromboembolic disease.

Etiopathogenesis

Pulmonary hypertension can be classified as follows:

Secondary Pulmonary Hypertension

1. *Increased pulmonary blood flow* leading to hyperkinetic PH occurs in congenital heart diseases with large left-to-right shunts like atrial septal defects, ventricular septal defects, and patent ductus arteriosus. PH occurs only when the pulmonary blood flow is increased 4–6 fold, thereby exceeding the reserve capacity of the pulmonary vascular bed.

2. a. *Increased resistance to pulmonary venous drainage (post-capillary PH)* leads to an increase in pulmonary

venous pressure which in turn causes passive increase in pulmonary artery pressure. It may be due to:

i. Elevated left ventricular diastolic pressure, e.g. left ventricular systolic dysfunction, reduced LV compliance, constrictive pericarditis. In fact, left ventricular failure is the most common cause of PH.

ii. Left atrial hypertension, e.g. in mitral valve disease, cor triatriatum, left atrial myxoma. Mitral stenosis is an important cause of PH. PH is initially due to left atrial hypertension (passive); subsequently pulmonary vasoconstriction occurs (reactive). Finally, anatomic changes may supervene (obstructive).

iii. Pulmonary venous obstruction, e.g. congenital stenosis of pulmonary veins, pulmonary venoocclusive disease, anomalous pulmonary venous connection with obstruction.

b. *Increased resistance to flow through the pulmonary vascular bed* is usually due to reduced cross-sectional area of the pulmonary vascular bed, as a result of chronic obstructive, restrictive or collagen-vascular disease of the lung. The predominant mechanism is perivascular parenchymal changes associated with pulmonary vasoconstriction due to hypoxia. Reduced cross-sectional area of the pulmonary vascular bed is also seen in persistent fetal circulation in the newborn.

c. *Increased resistance to flow through large pulmonary arteries*: Pulmonary embolism (common), peripheral pulmonic stenosis and unilateral absence or stenosis of a pulmonary artery (uncommon cause) constitute important causes.

3. *Hypoventilation*: Hypoxia and acidemia associated with hypoventilation cause vasoconstrictive or reactive PH due to constriction of small muscular pulmonary arteries and arterioles. This is seen in obesity-hypoventilation syndromes (Pickwickian syndrome), pharyngeal-tracheal obstruction and various neuromuscular and chest wall disorders.

4. *Miscellaneous causes*: The important ones are residence at high altitude, intravenous drug abuse and Takayasu's disease.

Primary Pulmonary Hypertension

Primary pulmonary hypertension (PPH), also referred to as essential, unexplained or idiopathic PH, is defined as pulmonary arterial hypertension of unknown cause. It is a diagnosis made by exclusion, by ruling out all recognizable causes of PH on the basis of clinical, electrocardiographic, radiological, echocardiographic and right-sided heart catheterization findings. The hemodynamic hallmark is a raised pulmonary artery pressure with normal or reduced cardiac output, and normal pulmonary wedge (left atrial) pressure. It is a disease commonly seen in young females.

The pathogenesis of PPH remains speculative. Histo-pathologic studies suggest that PPH is a disease of predisposed individuals and occurs as a result of exposure to various triggers of pulmonary vasoconstriction, leading to the development of characteristic vascular lesions, viz. plexiform lesions, angiomatoid lesions, concentric intimal fibrosis and necrotizing arteritis. The seat of the disease is the endothelium. An imbalance between vasoconstrictor-vasodilator mediators leads to release of thromboxane which causes platelet aggregation and vasoconstriction. Thrombosis in situ and smooth muscle cell proliferation also occur, resulting in reduced cross-sectional area of the pulmonary vascular bed and hence PH.

Clinical Features

Symptoms: The symptoms due to PH *per se* are exertional dyspnea, exhaustion, syncope and precordial pain. These are usually due to low cardiac output, hypoxia or both. Precordial pain is due to right ventricular ischemia or distension of major pulmonary arteries. Palpitations occur due to tachyarrhythmias. Rupture of plexiform lesion or pulmonary emboli may cause hemoptysis.

Signs: Physical examination reveals a prominent 'a' wave in the jugular venous pulse, low-volume carotid pulse with normal upstroke, right ventricular heave, systolic pulsations caused by the dilated pulmonary artery in the second left intercostal space, loud pulmonary component of the second heart sound, right-sided S_4 and systolic ejection click. Later, a right ventricular third heart sound, signs of pulmonary and tricuspid incompetence, cyanosis and congestive heart failure appear.

Investigations

The gold standard for the diagnosis of PH is right-sided heart catheterization. Noninvasive tests, as a rule, are less reliable and less informative. The electrocardiogram may show P pulmonale in leads II, III, aVF, right axis deviation, right ventricular hypertrophy and T inversion with ST depression in V_1–V_3. Chest X-ray shows a large main pulmonary artery and its major branches with attenuated peripheral pulmonary arteries. Right atrial and right ventricular enlargement may also be present (Table 12.1).

Table 12.1: Investigative approach to causes of pulmonary hypertension

Causes	Diagnostic studies	Result
1. Congenital heart disease	Cardiac catheterization, 2D echo	L to R and R to L shunts
2. Left sided lesions	2D echo, cardiac catheterization	Pulmonary wedge pressure increased
3. Pulmonary artery disease a. Major pulmonary artery occlusion	Pulmonary arterial pressure and angiography	Pressure gradients; stenosis or filling defects
b. Peripheral pulmonary artery stenosis c. Pulmonary embolic disease	Ventilation-perfusion scan	Abnormal
	Lung biopsy	Eccentric intimal fibrosis, fibrous strands
4. Pulmonary venous thrombosis or obstruction	X-ray chest, angiography, lung biopsy	Pulmonary vein changes
5. Pulmonary parenchymal disease	X-ray chest, pulmonary function studies, lung biopsy	
6. Collagen disease	LE cell, skin, muscle or lung biopsy	Perivascular inflammation

Treatment

The classification of treatment is shown in Table 12.2.

Table 12.2: Classification of treatment

A.	Curative
B.	Palliative
	a. Decrease resistance to pulmonary blood flow 　　1. Reduction of raised LV diastolic pressure 　　2. Pulmonary vasodilators 　　3. Anticoagulation 　　4. Oxygen therapy 　　5. Heart-lung transplantation
	b. Improve cardiocirculatory response to RV overload 　　1. Maximize alveolar ventilation and oxygenation by pulmonary toilet 　　2. Vaccine prophylaxis and prompt treatment for respiratory infection 　　3. Pulmonary vasodilator; management of cardiac failure

Curative

Treatment is curative only when it is possible to identify the underlying cause and correct it before irreversible damage has been done to the pulmonary vasculature; for example, surgical correction of congenital left-to-right shunts, mitral stenosis, cor triatriatum, left atrial myxoma, constrictive pericarditis, total anomalous pulmonary venous connection with obstruction, massively hypertrophied tonsils and adenoids will correct PH. Avoidance of the offending agent or drug is also useful.

There is no cure for primary PH nor is there a therapeutic approach that is uniformly accepted. However, due to improvement in the drug therapy for this disease, sustained clinical improvement and increased life expectancy can be expected in a substantial segment of this patient population.

The goal of vasodilator therapy is to reduce pulmonary artery pressure and increase cardiac output without symptomatic systemic hypotension. There is no selective pulmonary vasodilator agent and there is a marked heterogeneity in individual responsiveness to the various agents. Vasodilators used include adrenergic blockers (phentolamine, tolazoline), b-adrenergic agonists (isoproterenol), hydralazine, diazoxide, nitrates, calcium-channel blocking agents, angiotensin-converting enzyme inhibitors, and arachidonic acid metabolites (prostacyclin, prostaglandin E1). Among these, drugs which hold great promise are calcium-channels blocking agents (nifedipine and diltiazem) and arachidonic acid metabolites.

Anticoagulation

This is indicated in PH due to recurrent pulmonary emboli. It is also indicated in patients with severe PH as these patients are at risk for thrombotic events due to their sedentary lifestyle, venous insufficiency and sluggish pulmonary blood flow.

Oxygen Therapy

Supplemental low-flow oxygen therapy is useful in certain circumstances, e.g. in patients with parenchymal lung disease, patients residing at high altitude (to obviate hypoxic vasoconstriction) and those who respond to acute oxygen inhalation by a drop in the pulmonary artery pressure during hemodynamic study.

Heart-lung and Lung Transplantation

In patients with PH progressing to the stage of right ventricular failure refractory to medical management, heart-lung transplantation has evolved as a viable option in specialized centers. Besides PPH, heart-lung transplantation has been increasingly used for Eisenmenger's syndrome, cystic fibrosis and COPD. The survival rate is 60 percent at 1 year. Single-lung transplantation has emerged as an alternative option.

Chronic Cor Pulmonale

Definition

Chronic cor pulmonale is the term applied to hypertrophy of the right ventricle with or without right-sided heart failure due to pulmonary hypertension resulting from disease affecting the function or structure of the lung, except when these pulmonary alterations are the result of diseases that primarily affect the left side of the heart.

Incidence

Data from hospitals in Agra and Delhi show an incidence of 17.1 and 16.5 percent of all cardiac cases while it is reported to be 3.5 percent at Vellore in Tamil Nadu. Extremely cold winters with smoke, fog, and crowding in ill ventilated rooms and very hot summers with dust storms with consequent increase in respiratory infections may be responsible for its high incidence in North India.

Chronic cor pulmonale is mostly seen in middle and old age. Males are affected twice as commonly as females. This is because chronic bronchitis, emphysema and pneumoconiosis are more common in males.

Predisposing Factors

Poverty and chronic cor pulmonale go hand in hand. Poverty leads to malnutrition, reduced resistance to disease, and overcrowding, with a high incidence and inadequate treatment of respiratory infections. Incomplete recovery results in residual lung damage. Early return to manual work after illness further contributes to the disability with resulting cardiac complications.

Pneumoconiosis (especially anthracosis and silicosis) is an important predisposing factor. Coal and stone dust, in the course of years, cause marked fibrosis and obliteration of small arteries of the lungs.

Pathogenesis

Chronic lung disease mainly affects the heart by producing pulmonary hypertension. Hypoxia is a strong vasoconstrictor of the pulmonary artery and its branches. Other factors of leading to pulmonary hypertension are:

1. Anatomic reduction of the pulmonary vascular bed, from rupture of alveolar walls and by fibrotic and thrombotic obliteration of the capillaries
2. Compression of pulmonary capillaries by high intraalveolar pressures, when there is air trapping.

The factors which contribute to the clinical picture of chronic cor pulmonale are shown in Table 12.3.

Table 12.3: Factors contributing to cor pulmonale

1. Polycythemia and increased blood volume due to hypoxemia
2. Impaired myocardial function due to hypoxemia
3. Peripheral vasodilation due to increased arterial carbon dioxide tension, producing a large pulse pressure and warm extremities
4. Cerebral vasodilatation due to increased arterial carbon dioxide tension, leading to raised cerebrospinal fluid pressure, papilloedema, confusion and tremors.

Pathology

The characteristic features are dilatation and hypertrophy of the right ventricle, dilatation of the main pulmonary artery and enlargement of the right atrium. When the heart fails, dilatation of the right ventricle occurs followed by tricuspid insufficiency and right atrial dilatation.

Clinical Features

Symptoms

Three stages are distinguishable in the life history of chronic pulmonary disease:

1. Uncomplicated chronic pulmonary disease
2. Compensated cor pulmonale
3. Decompensated cor pulmonale with evidence of right heart failure.

Chronic cor pulmonale produces cardiac symptoms only when the heart begins to fail. During the stage of compensated cor pulmonale, the symptoms reflect the underlying pulmonary disease. The cardiac changes are detected only on investigation.

When pulmonary hypertension and right ventricular hypertrophy supervene and compensated chronic cor pulmonale develops, exertional dyspnea may be more pronounced, with dyspnea at rest and cyanosis especially during periods of exacerbation of pulmonary disease or with pulmonary infections.

Decompensated cor pulmonale is characterized by the presence of evidence of right heart failure with liver enlargement, systemic venous congestion and peripheral edema. Dyspnea and cyanosis are further intensified and along with the plethoric appearance and edema present a picture of so-called "blue bloaters".

Physical Signs

There may be little or no physical signs in the initial stages. Central cyanosis is variable. The extremities are usually warm. Capillary pulsation may be present in the pulp of the fingers. Papilloedema may be present. There may be signs of emphysema with restricted chest movements, barrel-shaped chest, harsh vesicular breath sounds with prolonged expiration, and rhonchi and crepitations in the lungs.

The features of right ventricular hypertrophy are generally masked by coexistent emphysema. The heart sounds are muffled. A right ventricular heave may be palpable in the epigastrium; pulmonary hypertension may be inferred from a loud pulmonary component of the second heart sound, an inconstant ejection click, an ejection systolic murmur in the 2nd and 3rd left intercostal spaces, and rarely a decrescendo diastolic murmur in the pulmonary area due to pulmonary regurgitation.

Signs of right heart failure may be present: Engorgement of neck veins, positive hepatojugular reflux, enlarged and tender liver, pitting edema in the dependent parts, right ventricular diastolic gallop and pansystolic murmur of tricuspid insufficiency.

Investigations

Investigations commonly carried out are shown in Table 12.4.

Table 12.4: Investigation of chronic cor pulmonale

• Hemoglobin
• Packed cell volume
• Total leukocyte count
• Differential leukocyte count
• Sputum examination
• Sputum culture and sensitivity
• Pulmonary function tests
• X-ray evaluation
• Electrocardiogram
• Hemodynamics

Electrocardiogram: The changes most commonly seen in chronic cor pulmonale are due to chronic obstructive emphysema exaggerated by the presence of right ventricular hypertrophy and dilatation (Fig. 12.1 and Table 12.5).

Chest X-ray: The earliest change is exaggeration of hilar shadows due to dilatation of the pulmonary artery and its branches resulting from pulmonary hypertension. With the onset of congestive heart failure, enlargement of right atrium and dilatation of superior vena cava are notable. Evidence of the underlying pulmonary disease is seen (Fig. 12.2).

Pulmonary function tests: Forced vital capacity (FVC) is reduced, but to a smaller extent than forced expiratory volume in the first second (FEV1). The residual volume is increased proportionately, the total lung volume remaining normal. Arterial blood gas analysis shows oxygen saturation ranging between 60 and 80 percent, reduction of PO_2 and a variable increase of PCO_2 especially in patients with underlying obstructive airway disease.

Diagnosis

Two types of diagnostic problems arise: (1) is the heart involved in a known case of chronic pulmonary disease? And (2) is right

Table 12.5: Electrocardiographic findings in chronic cor pulmonale

• Tall peaked P waves (P pulmonale) in leads L_2, L_3 and aVF with P_2 higher than P_1; P negative or flat in L_1 and aVL and often diphasic in V_1 and V_1
• Marked right axis deviation (1100 or more)
• Shift of the transitional zones to the left with persistence of S wave in V_5 and V_6
• S_1 S_2 S_3 syndrome characterized by prominent S wave in three standard limb leads without any prolongation of QRS interval with a small R' deflection in V_1. Cause of this type of change is right ventricular hypertrophy
• Inverted T waves in right precordial leads V_1–V_4 and also in leads L_3 and aVF
• Presence of qR pattern with late intrinsicoid deflection (more than 0.035 sec) in V_1, V_3R and V_4R. Incomplete right bundle branch block pattern (QRS less than 0.12 sec) may be present
• QRS complexes may be of low voltage especially over the precordial leads

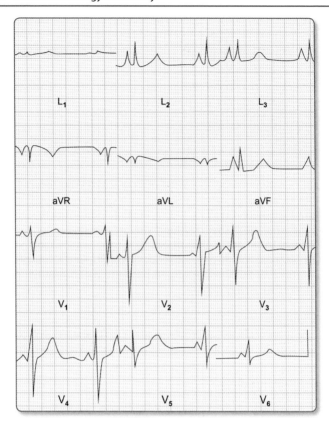

Fig. 12.1: Electrocardiogram showing tall P wave in L_2, L_3 and avF (P pulmonale), persistence of S wave in lead V_5, V_6 and right ventricular hypertrophy

sided heart failure due to pulmonary disease or to some other cause? The diagnosis of cor pulmonale requires demonstration of right ventricular hypertrophy by an electrocardiogram and a right ventricular third heard sound. Pulmonary function tests and blood gas studies evaluate the pulmonary disorder. In some patients echocardiography and hemodynamic and angiographic studies may be required.

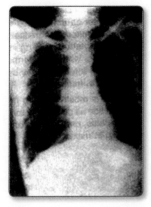

Fig. 12.2: Roentgenogram showing emphysema and chronic cor pulmonale. The heart is not enlarged but the pulmonary artery is prominent

Course and Prognosis

Chronic cor pulmonale begins insidiously, and despite the presence of distressing and sometimes disabling symptoms, a near normal lifespan is possible if recurrent respiratory infections are adequately treated. The onset of cardiac failure makes the prognosis poor. Treatment may alleviate an individual episode of heart failure but recurrent pulmonary infections precipitate further episodes of congestive heart failure which respond poorly to treatment, with the patients not likely to survive for long.

Another complication and at times a terminal event is the progressive increase of PCO_2 leading to carbon dioxide narcosis. It is precipitated in many patients by pulmonary infection, administration of sedatives or tranquilizers, and inadvertent continuous oxygen inhalation which depresses the respiratory center response by removing the hypoxic drive, leading to depressed respiration and accumulation of carbon dioxide.

Treatment

Smoking, poverty and air pollution are undoubtedly of great importance as predisposing factors in chronic cor pulmonale. Every attempt should be made to remedy the latter by industrial and social safeguards. Individuals must quit smoking. Vigorous preventive and symptomatic treatment of bronchitis and asthma may delay the development of serious emphysema and cor pulmonale. Early and energetic treatment of respiratory infections is mandatory to prevent or delay the onset of congestive heart failure.

Congestive heart failure requires treatment of any associated respiratory infection, correction of hypoxemia, reduction of carbon dioxide retention, relief of airway obstruction and management of heart failure.

Oxygen therapy is essential but should be cautiously used since a high concentration may lead to carbon dioxide retention and coma. Oxygen may be administered intermittently through a venturi mask designed to deliver 24 percent oxygen, enough to reduce life-threatening hypoxia while maintaining the hypoxic respiratory drive. In those with severe respiratory depression and respiratory failure, intermittent positive pressure breathing with a respirator is required.

In patients with cor pulmonale secondary to chronic obstructive pulmonary disease, long-term oxygen therapy at home can considerably enhance the quality of life as well as prolong life expectancy by several years.

Venesection as a therapeutic measure is controversial and is contraindicated in acute respiratory failure. However, in the presence of severe peripheral venous congestion with a high hematocrit and increased plasma volume, venesection may be rarely resorted to with caution.

Diuretics and low sodium intake are effective for controlling congestive heart failure. Digitalis should be used with caution in chronic cor pulmonale. It should preferably be avoided as digitalis toxicity is very common. Furosemide is useful as a diuretic; the dose is regulated according to the edema and severity of heart failure, and supplemented with potassium salts. After relief of heart failure, the patient should be instructed to avoid a dusty atmosphere and stop smoking. Respiratory infections must be promptly and adequately treated and obesity if present is corrected.

Pulmonary Embolism

Introduction

Background

Pulmonary embolism (PE) is a common and potentially lethal condition. Most patients who succumb to pulmonary embolism do so within the first few hours of the event. In patients who survive, recurrent embolism and death can be prevented with prompt diagnosis and therapy. Unfortunately, the diagnosis is often missed because patients with pulmonary embolism present with nonspecific signs and symptoms. If left untreated, approximately one-third of patients who survive an initial pulmonary embolism die from a subsequent embolic episode (Fig. 12.3).

The most important conceptual advance regarding pulmonary embolism over the last several decades has been the realization that pulmonary embolism is not a disease; rather, pulmonary embolism is a complication of venous thromboembolism, most commonly deep venous thrombosis (DVT).

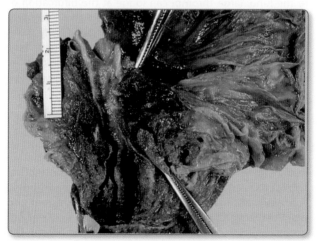

Fig. 12.3: Postmortem specimen of a large pulmonary artery thrombus in a hospitalized patient who died suddenly

Pathophysiology
Natural History of Venous Thrombosis

In the 19th century, Virchow identified a *triad of factors that lead to venous thrombosis*: Venous stasis, injury to the intima, and enhanced coagulation properties of the blood. Thrombosis usually originates as a platelet nidus on valves in the veins of the lower extremities. Further growth occurs by accretion of platelets and fibrin and progression to red fibrin thrombus, which may either break off and embolize or result in total occlusion of the vein. The endogenous thrombolytic system leads to partial dissolution; then, the thrombus becomes organized and is incorporated into the venous wall.

Natural History of Pulmonary Embolism

Pulmonary emboli usually arise from the thrombi originating in the deep venous system of the lower extremities; however, rarely they may originate in the pelvic, renal, or upper extremity veins or the right heart chambers. After traveling to the lung, large thrombi can lodge at the bifurcation of the main pulmonary artery or the lobar branches and cause hemodynamic compromise. Smaller thrombi typically travel more distally, occluding smaller vessels in the lung periphery. These are more likely to produce pleuritic chest pain by initiating an inflammatory response adjacent to the parietal pleura. Most pulmonary emboli are multiple, and the lower lobes are involved more commonly than the upper lobes.

Respiratory Consequences

Acute respiratory consequences of pulmonary embolism include increased alveolar dead space, pneumoconstriction, hypoxemia, and hyperventilation. Later, two additional consequences may occur: regional loss of surfactant and pulmonary infarction. Arterial hypoxemia is a frequent but not universal finding in patients with acute embolism. The mechanisms of hypoxemia include ventilation-perfusion mismatch, intrapulmonary shunts, reduced cardiac output, and intracardiac shunt via a patent foramen ovale. Pulmonary infarction is an uncommon consequence because of the bronchial arterial collateral circulation.

Hemodynamic Consequences

Pulmonary embolism reduces the cross-sectional area of the pulmonary vascular bed, resulting in an increment in pulmonary vascular resistance, which, in turn, increases the right ventricular afterload. If the afterload is increased severely, right ventricular failure may ensue. In addition, the humoral and reflex mechanisms contribute to the pulmonary arterial constriction. Prior poor cardiopulmonary status of the patient is an important factor leading to hemodynamic collapse. Following the initiation of anticoagulant therapy, the resolution of emboli occurs rapidly during the first 2 weeks of therapy. Significant long-term nonresolution of emboli causing pulmonary hypertension or cardiopulmonary symptoms is uncommon.

Frequency

The incidence of pulmonary embolism in the United States is estimated at 1 case per 1,000 persons per year.

Pulmonary embolism is present in 60–80 percent of patients with DVT, even though more than half these patients are asymptomatic. Pulmonary embolism is the third most common cause of death in hospitalized patients, with at least 650,000 cases occurring annually. Autopsy studies have shown that approximately 60 percent of patients who died in the hospital had pulmonary embolism, and the diagnosis was missed in upto 70 percent of the cases. Prospective studies have demonstrated DVT in 10–13 percent of all medical patients placed on bed rest for 1 week, 29–33 percent of all patients in medical intensive care units, 20–26 percent of patients with pulmonary diseases who are given bed rest for 3 or more days, 27–33 percent of those admitted to a critical care unit after a myocardial infarction, and 48 percent of patients who are asymptomatic after a coronary artery bypass graft.

Among postpartum women, the annual incidence was 5 times higher than in pregnant women.

Mortality/Morbidity

As a cause of sudden death, massive pulmonary embolism is second only to sudden cardiac death. Autopsy studies of patients who died unexpectedly in a hospital setting have shown approximately 80 percent of these patients died from massive pulmonary embolism.

Approximately 10 percent of patients who develop pulmonary embolism die within the first hour, and 30 percent die subsequently from recurrent embolism. Anticoagulant treatment decreases the mortality rate to less than 5 percent. The diagnosis of pulmonary embolism is missed in approximately 400,000 patients in the United States per year; approximately 100,000 deaths could be prevented with proper diagnosis and treatment.

Race

The incidence of and mortality rates from pulmonary embolism appears to be significantly higher in blacks than in whites. Mortality rates for whites have been 50 percent higher than those for people of other races (e.g. Asians, Native Americans).

Sex

The risk of pulmonary embolism is increased in pregnancy and during the postpartum period. The death rates from pulmonary embolism were 20–30 percent higher among men than among women.

Age

In hospitalized elderly patients, pulmonary embolism is commonly missed and often is the cause of death. It can occur at any age in a bedridden or immobile (say due to fracture or paralysis) patient.

Clinical Symptoms

- The symptoms of pulmonary embolism are nonspecific; therefore, a high index of suspicion is required, particularly when a patient has risk factors for the condition (see Causes, page 209).

The most common symptoms of pulmonary embolism are dyspnea (73%), pleuritic chest pain (66%), cough (37%), and hemoptysis (13%). However, patients with pulmonary embolism may present with atypical symptoms. These symptoms include the following:

- Seizures
- Syncope
- Abdominal pain
- Fever
- Productive cough
- Wheezing
- Decreasing level of consciousness
- New onset of atrial fibrillation
- Flank pain
- Delirium (in elderly patients).

Pleuritic chest pain without other symptoms or risk factors may be a presentation of pulmonary embolism.

The diagnosis of pulmonary embolism should be sought actively in patients with respiratory symptoms unexplained by an alternate diagnosis. The presentation of patients with pulmonary embolism can be categorized into 4 classes based on the acuity and severity of pulmonary arterial occlusion:

1. Massive pulmonary embolism: Large emboli compromise sufficient pulmonary circulation to produce circulatory collapse and shock. The patient has hypotension; appears weak, pale, sweaty, and oliguric; and develops impaired mentation.
2. Acute pulmonary infarction: In Approximately 10 percent of patients there is peripheral occlusion of a pulmonary artery causing parenchymal infarction. These patients present with acute onset of pleuritic chest pain, breathlessness, and hemoptysis. Although the chest pain may be clinically indistinguishable from ischemic myocardial pain, normal electrocardiogram findings and no response to nitroglycerin rules it out.
3. Acute embolism without infarction: Patients have non-specific symptoms of unexplained dyspnea and/or substernal discomfort.

4. Multiple pulmonary emboli. (a) Repeated documented episodes of pulmonary emboli over years, eventually presenting with signs and symptoms of pulmonary hypertension and cor pulmonale. (b) No previously documented pulmonary emboli but have widespread obstruction of the pulmonary circulation with clot. They present with gradually progressive dyspnea, intermittent exertional chest pain, and, eventually, features of pulmonary hypertension and cor pulmonale.

Most patients with pulmonary embolism have no obvious symptoms at presentation. In contrast, patients with symptomatic DVT commonly have pulmonary embolism confirmed on diagnostic studies in the absence of pulmonary symptoms.

Signs

The most common physical signs are as follows:

- Tachypnea (70%)
- Rales (51%)
- Tachycardia (30%)
- Fourth heart sound (24%)
- Accentuated pulmonic component of the second heart sound (23%).

Fever of less than 39°C may be present in 14 percent of patients; however, temperature higher than 39.5°C is not from pulmonary embolism. Finally, chest wall tenderness upon palpation, without a history of trauma, may be the sole physical finding in rare cases.

Physical examination findings are quite variable in pulmonary embolism and, for convenience, may be grouped into four categories as follows:

1. *Massive pulmonary embolism*: These patients are in shock: Systemic hypotension, poor perfusion of the extremities, tachycardia, and tachypnea. Additionally, signs of pulmonary hypertension such as palpable impulse over the second left intercostal space, loud P_2, right ventricular S_3 gallop, and a systolic murmur louder on inspiration at left sternal border (tricuspid regurgitation) may be present. Signs of pleural

effusion, such as dullness to percussion and diminished breath sounds, may be present

2. *Acute embolism without infarction*: These patients have nonspecific physical signs that may easily be secondary to another disease process: Tachypnea and tachycardia frequently are detected, pleuritic pain sometimes may be present, crackles may be heard in the area of embolization, and local wheeze may be heard rarely.

3. *Multiple pulmonary emboli or thrombi*: Patients belonging to both the subsets in this category have physical signs of pulmonary hypertension and cor pulmonale: Elevated jugular venous pressure, right ventricular heave, palpable impulse in the left second intercostal space, right ventricular S_3 gallop, systolic murmur over the left sternal border that is louder during inspiration, hepatomegaly, ascites, and dependent pitting edema. These findings are not specific for pulmonary embolism and require a high index of suspicion for pursuing appropriate diagnostic studies.

Causes

The causes for pulmonary embolism are multifactorial and are not readily apparent in many cases. The following causes have been described in the literature:

1. *Venous stasis*: Increased viscosity may occur due to polycythemia and dehydration, immobility, raised venous pressure in cardiac failure, or compression of a vein by a tumor.

2. *Hypercoagulable states*:
   – Factor V Leiden mutation causing resistance to activated protein C is the most common cause of familial thromboembolism (5% of population)
   – Primary or acquired deficiencies in protein C, protein S, and antithrombin III are other risk factors. The deficiency of these natural anticoagulants is responsible for 10 percent of venous thrombosis in younger people

3. Immobilization
   – Prolonged bed rest or immobilization of a limb in a cast
   – Paralysis increases the risk

4. Surgery and trauma
   - Both surgical and accidental traumas predispose patients to venous thromboembolism by activating clotting factors and causing immobility
   - Fractures of the femur and tibia are associated with the highest risk, followed by pelvic, spinal, and other fractures
   - Severe burns carry a high risk of DVT or pulmonary embolism
   - Pulmonary embolism may account for 15 percent of all postoperative deaths. Leg amputations and hip, pelvic, and spinal surgery are associated with the highest risk
5. Pregnancy
   - The mechanism of DVT is venous stasis, decreasing fibrinolytic activity, and increased procoagulant factors.
6. Oral contraceptives and estrogen replacement
   - Estrogen-containing birth control pills have increased the occurrence of venous thromboembolism in healthy women.
   - The risk is proportional to the estrogen content and is increased in postmenopausal women on hormonal replacement therapy (HRT)
   - The relative risk is 3-fold.
7. Malignancy
   - Malignancy has been identified in 17 percent of patients with venous thromboembolism.

Immobilization (usually because of surgery) is the risk factor most commonly assessed in patients with pulmonary embolism; 94 percent of all patients with pulmonary embolism have 1 or more of the following risk factors:

- Immobilization
- Travel of 4 hour or more in the past month
- Surgery within the last 3 months
- Malignancy, especially lung cancer
- Current or past history of thrombophlebitis
- Trauma to the lower extremities and pelvis during the past 3 months
- Smoking

- Central venous instrumentation within the past 3 months
- Stroke, paresis, or paralysis
- Prior pulmonary embolism
- Heart failure
- Chronic obstructive pulmonary disease.

Other recognized risk factors include the following:

- Obesity
- Varicose veins
- Inflammatory bowel disease.

Differential Diagnoses

Differential diagnoses are extensive, and they should be considered carefully with any patient thought to have pulmonary embolism. These patients also should have an alternate diagnosis confirmed, or pulmonary embolism should be excluded, before discontinuing the workup. Problems to be considered include the following: IHD, pleuritic pain, fat embolism, musculoskeletal pain, costochondritis, rib fracture, pericarditis, angina pectoris, salicylate intoxication, hyperventilation.

Investigations

1. D-dimer testing
   - Negative results on a high-sensitivity D-dimer test in a patient indicate a low likelihood of venous thromboembolism and reliably exclude pulmonary embolism. D-dimer testing is most reliable for excluding pulmonary embolism in younger patients who have no associated comorbidity or history of venous thromboembolism and whose symptoms are of short duration. D-dimer testing is of questionable value in patients who are older than 80 years, are hospitalized, or have cancer and in pregnant women, because nonspecific elevation of D-dimer concentrations is common in such patients. D-dimer test should not be used when the clinical probability of pulmonary embolism is high, because the test has low negative predictive value in such cases (Fig. 12.4).

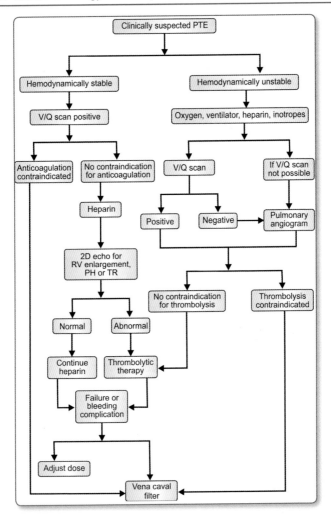

Fig. 12.4: Algorithm for management of clinically suspected PTE. HD = hemodynamically, RV-right ventricular, PH = pulmonary hypertension, TR = tricuspid regurgitation, V/Q = ventilation-perfusion

- Arterial blood gases
  - Arterial blood gas determinations characteristically reveal hypoxemia, hypocapnia, and respiratory alkalosis; however, the predictive value of hypoxemia is quite low.

Imaging Studies

- Chest radiography
  - This is the most appropriate study for ruling out other causes of chest pain in patients with suspected pulmonary embolism.
  - Initially, the chest radiography findings are normal in most cases of pulmonary embolism. However, in later stages, radiographic signs may include a Westermark sign (dilatation of pulmonary vessels and a sharp cutoff), atelectasis, a small pleural effusion, and an elevated diaphragm (Figs 12.5 and 12.6).

Computed Tomography

Computed tomography angiography (CTA) is the initial imaging modality of choice for stable patients with suspected pulmonary

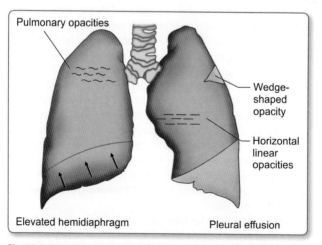

Fig. 12.5: Diagrammatic representation of radiological features of pulmonary thromboembolism

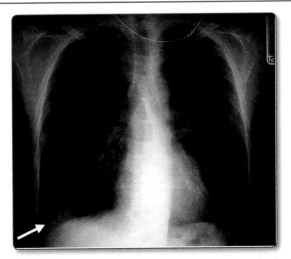

Fig. 12.6: A posteroanterior chest radiograph showing a peripheral wedge-shaped infiltrate caused by pulmonary infarction secondary to pulmonary embolism. Hampton hump is a rare and nonspecific finding

embolism. In patients with a negative CTA, the likelihood for subsequent thromboembolic events is extremely small.

Spiral CT can visualize main, lobar, and segmental pulmonary emboli with a reported sensitivity of greater than 90 percent. Spiral CT scanning can help detect emboli as small as 2 mm that are affecting upto the seventh border division of the pulmonary artery. A significant limitation of spiral CT scanning is that small subsegmental emboli may not be detected (Figs 12.7 to 12.12).

- *Ventilation-perfusion (V/Q) scanning of the lungs*: This is an important diagnostic modality for establishing the diagnosis of pulmonary embolism. However, V/Q scanning should be used only when CT scanning is not available or if the patient has a contraindication to CT scanning or intravenous contrast material.
- Noninvasive tests for lower extremity DVT
  - These may be helpful in the evaluation of patients who have nondiagnostic V/Q scan patterns of intermediate and low probability.

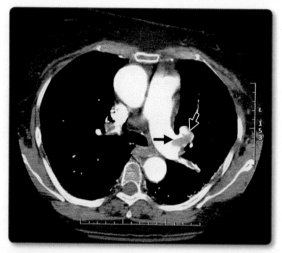

Fig. 12.7: A spiral CT scan shows thrombus in bilateral main pulmonary arteries

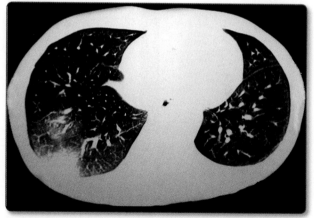

Fig. 12.8: CT scan of the same chest depicted in previous image

- Pulmonary angiography
  - Pulmonary angiography remains the criterion standard for the diagnosis of pulmonary embolism.

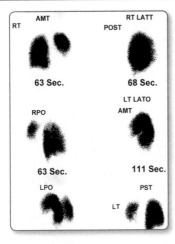

Fig. 12.9: High-probability perfusion lung scan shows segmental perfusion defects in the right upper lobe and subsegmental perfusion defects in right lower lobe, left upper lobe, and left lower lobe

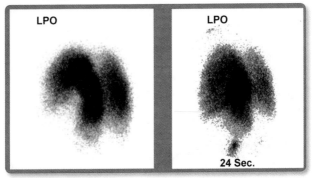

Fig. 12.10: A segmental ventilation perfusion mismatch evident in a left anterior oblique projection

- Positive results consist of a filling defect or sharp cutoff of the affected artery. Nonocclusive emboli are described to have a tram-track appearance.
- Negative pulmonary angiogram findings, even if false-negative, exclude clinically relevant pulmonary embolism.

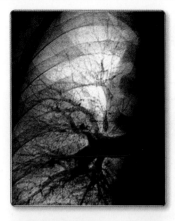

Fig. 12.11: A pulmonary angiogram shows the abrupt termination of the ascending branch of the right upperlobe artery, confirming the diagnosis of pulmonary embolism

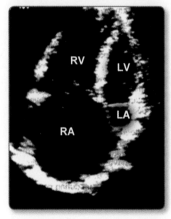

Fig. 12.12: Apical four-chamber echocardiogram in massive pulmonary embolism showing a dilated right ventricle (RV) and a dilated right atrium (RA). LA - left atrium, LV - left ventricle

- Magnetic resonance imaging
  - Pulmonary emboli demonstrate increased signal intensity within the pulmonary artery. By obtaining a sequence of images, this signal that is originating from slow blood flow may be distinguished from pulmonary embolism.
- Echocardiography
  This modality generally has limited accuracy in the diagnosis of pulmonary embolism.

Echocardiography may demonstrate right ventricular dysfunction in acute pulmonary embolism, predicting a higher mortality and possible benefit from thrombolytic therapy (Fig. 12.13).

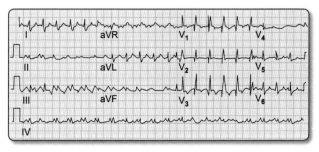

Fig. 12.13: Echocardiography shows right ventricular dysfunction in acute pulmonary embolism

Other Tests

Electrocardiography: The most common ECG abnormalities of pulmonary embolism are tachycardia and nonspecific ST-T wave abnormalities. These findings are not sensitive or specific enough to aid in the diagnosis of pulmonary embolism. The classic finding of right-sided heart strain demonstrated by an S1-Q3-T3 pattern is observed in only 20 percent of patients with proven pulmonary embolism.

Treatment

Medical Care

Immediate full anticoagulation is mandatory for all patients suspected to have deep vein thrombosis (DVT) or pulmonary embolism (PE). Current guidelines recommend starting unfractionated heparin (UFH), low molecular weight heparin (LMWH) or fondaparinux in addition to an oral anticoagulant (warfarin) at the time of diagnosis, and to discontinue UH, LMWH, or fondaparinux only after the international normalized ratio (INR) is 2.0 for at least 24 hours, but no sooner than 5 days after warfarin therapy has been started.

Thrombolytic therapy: Thrombolytic therapy should be considered for patients who are hemodynamically unstable, patients who have right-sided heart strain, and high-risk patients with underlying poor cardiopulmonary reserve (Table 12.6).

Although most studies demonstrate superiority of thrombolytic therapy with respect to resolution of radiographic and hemodynamic abnormalities within the first 24 hours, this advantage disappears 7 days after treatment. Controlled clinical trials have not demonstrated benefit in terms of reduced mortality rates or earlier resolution of symptoms when currently compared with heparin.

- Goals of anticoagulation therapy

  The efficacy of heparin therapy depends on achieving a critical therapeutic level of heparin within the first 24 hours of treatment. The critical therapeutic level of heparin is 1.5 times the baseline control value or the upper limit of normal range of the activated partial thromboplastin time (aPTT).

  - If intravenous UFH is chosen, an initial bolus of 80 U/kg or 5000 U followed by an infusion of 18 U/kg/h or 1300 U/h should be given, with the goal of rapidly achieving and maintaining the aPTT at levels that correspond to therapeutic heparin levels.

- Low molecular weight heparin

  - Current guidelines for patients with acute nonmassive pulmonary embolism recommend LMWH over UFH (grade 1A). In patients with massive pulmonary embolism, if concerns regarding subcutaneous absorption arise, severe renal failure exists, or if thrombolytic therapy is being considered, intravenous UFH is the recommended form of initial anticoagulation (grade 2C).

Table 12.6: Thrombolytic therapy regimens for PTE

• Streptokinase	250,000 U IV (loading dose over 30 min), followed by 100,000 U/h for 24 hours
• Urokinase	4400 IU/kg IV (loading dose over 20 min), followed by 4400 IU/kg/h for 12 hours
• Tissue-type	100 mg (56 million IU) IV over 2 hours plasminogen activator

LMWHs have many advantages over UFH. These agents have a greater bioavailability, can be administered by subcutaneous injections, and have a longer duration of anticoagulant effect. A fixed dose of LMWH can be used, and laboratory monitoring of aPTT is not necessary.

Trials comparing LMWH with UFH have shown that LMWH is at least as effective and as safe as UFH.

LMWH can be administered safely in an outpatient setting.

Fondaparinux
- Fondaparinux is a synthetic polysaccharide derived from the antithrombin binding region of heparin. Fondaparinux catalyzes factor Xa inactivation by antithrombin without inhibiting thrombin.
- With the exception of patients presenting with massive pulmonary embolism (defined by hemodynamic compromise), LMWH or fondaparinux is recommended over intravenous UFH. This is because of a more predictable bioavailability, more rapid onset of full anticoagulant effect, and benefit of not typically needing to monitor anticoagulant effect.
- However, in cases in which an anticoagulant with a shorter half-life is more desirable (i.e. patients at particularly high risk of bleeding) or in patients with impaired renal function, intravenous UFH may be preferred.

Oral Anticoagulant Therapy
- The anticoagulant effect of warfarin is mediated by the inhibition of vitamin K dependent factors, which are II, VII, IX, and X. The peak effect does not occur until 36–72 hours after drug administration, and the dosage is difficult to titrate.
- A prothrombin time ratio is expressed as an INR and is monitored to assess the adequacy of warfarin therapy. The recommended therapeutic range for venous thromboembolism is an INR of 2–3. This level of anticoagulation markedly reduces the risk of bleeding without the loss of effectiveness. Initially, INR measurements are performed on a daily basis; once the patient is stabilized on a specific dose

of warfarin, the INR determinations may be performed every 1–2 weeks or at longer intervals.

Duration of anticoagulation
- A patient with a first thromboembolic event occurring in the setting of reversible risk factors such as immobilization, surgery, or trauma, should receive warfarin therapy for at least 3 months. Among patients with idiopathic (or unprovoked) first events. The current recommendation is anticoagulation for at least 3 months.
- Warfarin treatment for longer than 6 months is indicated in patients with recurrent venous thromboembolism or in those in whom a continuing risk factor for venous thromboembolism exists, including malignancy, immobilization, or morbid obesity.
- Patients who have pulmonary embolism and preexisting irreversible risk factors, such as deficiency of antithrombin III, protein S and C, factor V Leiden mutation, or the presence of antiphospholipid antibodies, should be placed on long-term anticoagulation.

Compression stockings: For patients who have had a proximal DVT, elastic compression stockings with a pressure of 30–40 mmHg at the ankle for 2 years following the diagnosis is recommended to reduce the risk of postphlebitic syndrome.

Surgical Care
The current grade 1A recommendation is that patients with acute pulmonary embolism should not routinely receive vena cava filters in addition to anticoagulants.

Inferior vena cava (IVC) interruption by the insertion of an IVC filter (Greenfield filter) is only indicated in the following settings:
- Patients with acute venous thromboembolism who have an absolute contraindication to anticoagulant therapy (e.g. recent surgery, hemorrhagic stroke, significant active or recent bleeding)

Patients with massive pulmonary embolism who survived but in whom recurrent embolism invariably will be fatal.

Activity

Activity is recommended as tolerated. Early ambulation is recommended over bed rest when feasible.

Follow-up
Prevention
Heparin prophylaxis

The incidence of venous thrombosis, pulmonary embolism (PE), and death can be significantly reduced by embracing a prophylactic strategy in high-risk patients (Table 12.7).

Table 12.7: Prophylaxis against venous thromboembolism

Condition	Risk (%)*	Recommendations
General Surgery		
Low risk	3	(1) Early ambulation
Moderate risk	29	(1) Unfractionated heparin: 5000 U SC given 2 hour preoperatively and q12h postoperatively (2) Dalteparin: 2500 U 1–2 hour before surgery, then once daily Enoxaparin: 2000 U before surgery, then once daily Nadroparin: 3100 U 2 hour before surgery, then once daily Tinzaparin: 3500 U 2 hour before surgery, then once daily
High-risk	39	(1) Unfractionated heparin: 5000 U SC given 2 hour preoperatively and q8h postoperatively (2) Dalteparin: 5000 U 10–12 hour before surgery, then once daily Enoxaparin: 4000 U 10–12 hour before surgery, then once daily
Very high-risk	80	(1) Unfractionated heparin: 5000 U SC given 2 hour preoperatively and q8h postoperatively; dalteparin: 2500 U given 2 hour preoperatively and qd; plus, intermittent pneumatic compression applied intraoperatively (2) Dalteparin: 5000 U 10–12 hour before surgery, then once daily Enoxaparin: 4000 U 10–12 hour before surgery, then once daily (3) Perioperative warfarin: INR 2–3

Contd...

Contd...

Orthopedic Surgery/Neurological Surgery/Trauma		
Total hip replacement	51	(1) Dalteparin: 5000 U 1–2 hour before surgery, then once daily Enoxaparin: 3000 U 10–12 hour before surgery, then once daily Nadroparin: 40 U/kg U 2 hour before surgery, then once daily Tinzaparin: 50 U/kg 2 hour before surgery, then 75 U/kg once daily (2) Warfarin: Preoperatively and adjusted to INR of 2–3 postoperatively, continue upto 4 week after surgery
Total knee replacement	61	(1) Dalteparin: 5000 U 1–2 hour before surgery, then once daily Enoxaparin: 3000 U 10–12 hour before surgery, then once daily Nadroparin: 40 U/kg U 2 hour before surgery, then once daily Tinzaparin: 50 U/kg 2 hour before surgery, then 75 U/kg once daily (2) Warfarin: Preoperatively and adjusted to INR of 2–3 postoperatively, continue upto 4 week after surgery
Hip fracture surgery	48	(1) Dalteparin: 5000 U 1–2 hour before surgery, then once daily Enoxaparin: 3000 U 10–12 hour before surgery, then once daily Nadroparin: 40 U/kg U 2 hour before surgery, then once daily Tinzaparin: 50 U/kg 2 hour before surgery, then 75 U/kg once daily (2) Warfarin: Preoperatively and adjusted to INR of 2–3 postoperatively, continue upto 4 week after surgery
Neurosurgery	24	(1) Intermittent pneumatic compression (2) Unfractionated heparin: 5000 U SC q12h and intermittent pneumatic compression for high-risk patients
Acute spinal cord injury with leg paralysis	40	(1) Unfractionated heparin: SC in doses adjusted to paralysis produce aPTT = 1.5 X control 6 h after dose (2) Enoxaparin: 3000 U twice daily (3) Warfarin: Adjusted to INR of 2–3 in rehabilitation phase (4) Intermittent pneumatic compression plus unfractionated heparin: 5000 U SC q12h

Contd...

Contd...

Multiple trauma	53	(1) Intermittent pneumatic compression until further bleeding is unlikely; then, give (2) Enoxaparin: 30 mg SC q12h or (3) Warfarin: Adjusted to INR of 2–3
Medical Conditions		
Acute myocardial infarction	24	Unfractionated heparin: 5000 U SC q12h unless therapeutic anticoagulation used
Ischemic stroke with paralysis	42	Unfractionated heparin: 5000 U SC q12h
Medical patients (cancer, bed rest, congestive heart failure, severe lung disease)	20	(1) Unfractionated heparin: 5000 U SC q12h (2) Dalteparin: 2500 U once daily Enoxaparin: 2000 U once daily

- Patients who have objectively documented recurrent venous thromboembolism, adequate anticoagulant therapy notwithstanding

*Approximate risk without prophylaxis for all and/or proximal DVT or symptomatic PE.

Sequential Compression Devices

Compression stockings provide a compression of 30–40 mmHg gradient and are a safe and effective therapy to prevent venous thromboembolism in patients who are at high-risk when heparin therapy is not desirable or is contraindicated. These devices provide a gradient of compression that is highest at the toes and gradually decreases to the level of the thigh. This mechanism reduces the capacitative venous volume by approximately 70 percent and increases the measured velocity of blood flow by a factor of 5 or more in lower extremity veins.

Complications

- Sudden cardiac death
- Obstructive shock
- Pulse less electrical activity

- Atrial or ventricular arrhythmias
- Secondary pulmonary arterial hypertension
- Cor pulmonale
- Severe hypoxemia
- Right-to-left intracardiac shunt
- Lung infarction
- Pleural effusion
- Paradoxical embolism.

Prognosis

- The prognosis of patients with pulmonary embolism depends on two factors: (1) the underlying disease state and (2) appropriate diagnosis and treatment.
- Most patients treated with anticoagulants do not develop long-term sequelae upon follow-up evaluation.
- At 5 days of anticoagulant therapy, 36 percent of lung scan defects are resolved; at 2 weeks, 52 percent are resolved; at 3 months, 73 percent are resolved.
- The mortality rate in patients with undiagnosed pulmonary embolism is 30 percent.
- The 1-year mortality rate is 24 percent. The deaths occur due to cardiac disease, recurrent pulmonary embolism, infection, and cancer.
- The risk of recurrent pulmonary embolism is due to the recurrence of proximal venous thrombosis; approximately 17 percent of patients with recurrent pulmonary embolism were found to have proximal DVT.
- In a small proportion of patients, pulmonary embolism does not resolve; hence, chronic thromboembolic pulmonary arterial hypertension results.

Special Concerns

- *Pregnancy:* The risk of venous thromboembolism is increased during pregnancy and the postpartum period. Pregnant women who are in a hypercoagulable state or have had previous venous thromboembolism should receive prophylactic anticoagulation during pregnancy.

Pregnant patients diagnosed with DVT or pulmonary embolism are treated with unfractionated heparin or LMWH throughout their pregnancy. Warfarin is contraindicated because it crosses the placental barrier and can cause fetal malformations. Therefore, either subcutaneous unfractionated heparin or LMWH at full anticoagulation doses should be continued until delivery. Women experiencing a thromboembolic event during pregnancy should receive therapeutic treatment with unfractionated heparin or LMWH during pregnancy, with anticoagulation continuing for 4–6 weeks postpartum, and for a total of at least 6 months.

- *Heparin-induced thrombocytopenia:* Heparin-induced thrombocytopenia (HIT) is a transient prothrombotic disorder initiated by heparin.
  Main features are (1) thrombocytopenia resulting from immunoglobulin G–mediated platelet activation and (2) in vivo thrombin generation and increased risk of venous and arterial thrombosis.

  The highest frequency of HIT, 5 percent, has been reported in postorthopedic surgery patients receiving upto 2 weeks of unfractionated heparin. HIT occurred in approximately 0.5 percent of postorthopedic surgery patients receiving LMWH for up to 2 weeks.

  HIT may manifest clinically as extension of the thrombus or formation of new arterial thrombosis. HIT should be suspected whenever the patient's platelet count falls to less than 100,000/µL or less than 50 percent of the baseline value, generally after 5–15 days of heparin therapy. The definitive diagnosis is made by performing a platelet activation factor assay.

  The treatment of patients who develop HIT is to stop all heparin products, including catheter flushes and heparin-coated catheters, and to initiate an alternative nonheparin anticoagulant, even when thrombosis is not clinically apparent. Preferred agents include direct thrombin inhibitors such as lepirudin or argatroban. Start warfarin while the patient receives an alternative nonheparin anticoagulant and only when the platelet count has recovered to at least 100,000/μL, preferably 150,000/μL.

- *Resistance to heparin:* Few patients with venous thromboembolism require large doses of heparin for achieving an optimal activated partial thromboplastin time (aPTT). These patients have increased plasma concentrations of factor VIII and heparin-binding proteins. Increased factor VIII concentration causes dissociation between aPTT and plasma heparin values. The aPTT is suboptimal, but patients have adequate heparin levels upon protamine titration. This commonly occurs in patients with a concomitant inflammatory disease.

  Monitoring the antifactor Xa assay results in this situation is safe and effective and results in less escalation of the heparin dose when compared with monitoring with aPTT. Whenever a therapeutic level of aPTT cannot be achieved with large doses of unfractionated heparin administration, either determination of plasma heparin concentration or therapy with LMWH should be instituted.

- *Elderly individuals:* Pulmonary embolism is increasingly prevalent among elderly patients, yet the diagnosis is missed more often in this population because respiratory symptoms often are dismissed as being chronic.

  Even when the diagnosis is made, appropriate therapy frequently is inappropriately withheld because of bleeding concerns.

  An appropriate diagnostic workup and therapeutic anticoagulation with a careful risk-to-benefit assessment is recommended in this patient population.

Thoracic Aortic Aneurysm

Introduction

Aneurysmal degeneration can occur anywhere in the human aorta. By definition, an aneurysm is a localized or diffuse dilation of an artery with a diameter at least 50 percent greater than the normal size of the artery.

True and False Aneurysms

Aneurysms are either true or false. The wall of a true aneurysm involves all three layers (intima, media, and adventitia) and the aneurysm is contained inside the endothelium. The wall of a false or pseudoaneurysm only involves the outer layer and is contained by the adventitia. An aortic dissection is formed by an intimal tear and is contained by the media; hence, it has a true lumen and a false lumen.

Most aortic aneurysms (AA) occur in the abdominal aorta; these are termed abdominal aortic aneurysms (AAA). Although most abdominal aortic aneurysms are asymptomatic at the time of diagnosis, the most common complication remains life-threatening rupture with hemorrhage.

Aneurysmal degeneration that occurs in the thoracic aorta is termed a thoracic aneurysm (TA). Aneurysms that coexist in both segments of the aorta (thoracic and abdominal) are termed thoracoabdominal aneurysms (TAA). Thoracic aneurysms and thoracoabdominal aneurysms are also at risk for rupture. Thoracic aortic aneurysms are subdivided into three groups depending on location: Ascending aortic, aortic arch, and descending thoracic aneurysms or thoracoabdominal aneurysms. Aneurysms that involve the ascending aorta may extend as proximally as the aortic annulus and as distally as the innominate artery, whereas descending thoracic aneurysms begin beyond the left subclavian artery. Arch aneurysms are as the name implies.

Dissection is another condition that may affect the thoracic aorta. An intimal tear causes separation of the walls of the aorta. A false passage for blood develops between the layers of the aorta. This false lumen may extend into branches of the aorta in the chest or abdomen, causing malperfusion, ischemia, or occlusion with resultant complications. The dissection can also progress proximally, to involve the aortic sinus, aortic valve, and coronary arteries. Dissection can lead to aneurysmal change and early or late rupture. A chronic dissection is one that is diagnosed more than 2 weeks after the onset of symptoms. Dissection should not be termed dissecting aneurysm because it can occur with or without aneurysmal enlargement of the aorta.

Fusiform and Saccular Aneurysms: The shape of an aortic aneurysm is either saccular or fusiform. A fusiform (or true) aneurysm has a uniform shape with a symmetrical dilatation that involves the entire circumference of the aortic wall. A saccular aneurysm is a localized out pouching of the aortic wall, and it is the shape of a pseudoaneurysm (Fig. 13.1).

Problem

Aneurysms are usually defined as a localized dilation of an arterial segment greater then 50 percent its normal diameter. Most aortic aneurysms occur in the infrarenal segment (95%).

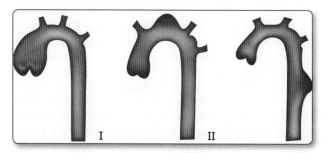

Fig. 13.1: Different types of aneurysms I. Fusiform aneurysm—usually ascending aorta II. Saccular aneurysms—arch of aorta or descending aorta

The average size for an infrarenal aorta is 2 cm; therefore, abdominal aortic aneurysms are usually defined by diameters greater than 3 cm.

The average diameter of the mid-descending thoracic aorta is 26–28 mm, compared with 20–23 mm at the level of the celiac axis.

Frequency

Although findings from autopsy series vary widely, the prevalence of aortic aneurysms probably exceeds 3–4 percent in individuals older than 65 years.

The estimated incidence of thoracic aortic aneurysms is 6 cases per 100,000 person-years. In addition, the overall prevalence of aortic aneurysms has increased significantly in the last 30 years.

Etiology

Aging results in changes in collagen and elastin, which lead to weakening of the aortic wall and aneurysmal dilation. Arteriosclerotic (degenerative) disease is the most common cause of thoracic aneurysms.

A previous aortic dissection with a persistent false channel may produce aneurysmal dilation; such aneurysms are the second most common type. False aneurysms are more common in the descending aorta and arise from the extravasation of blood into a tenuous pocket contained by the aortic adventitia. Because of increasing wall stress, false aneurysms tend to enlarge over time.

Authorities strongly agree that genetics play a role in the formation of aortic aneurysms. Of first-degree relatives of patients with aortic aneurysms, 15 percent have an aneurysm.

Individuals with Marfan's syndrome are at risk for aneurysmal degeneration, especially in the thoracic aorta.

Type IV Ehlers-Danlos syndrome results in a deficiency in the production of type III collagen, and individuals with this disease may develop aneurysms in any portion of the aorta.

Atherosclerosis may play a role. Other causes of aortic aneurysms are infection (i.e. bacterial [mycotic or syphilitic]), arteritis (i.e. giant cell, Takayasu's, Kawasaki, Behçet), and trauma.

Traumatic dissection is a result of shearing from deceleration injury due to high speed motor vehicle accidents (MVA) or a fall from heights. The dissection occurs at a point of fixation, usually at the aortic isthmus (i.e. at the ligamentum arteriosum, distal to the origin of the left subclavian artery), the ascending aorta, the aortic root, and the diaphragmatic hiatus.

The true etiology of aortic aneurysms is probably multi-factorial, and the condition occurs in individuals with multiple risk factors. Risk factors include smoking, chronic obstructive pulmonary disease (COPD), hypertension, atherosclerosis, male gender, older age, high BMI, bicuspid or unicuspid aortic valves, genetic disorders, and family history. Aortic aneurysms are more common in men than in women and are more common in persons with COPD than in those without lung disease.

Presentation

1. Most patients with aortic aneurysms are asymptomatic at the time of discovery. Thoracic aneurysms are usually found incidentally after chest radiographs or other imaging studies.

2. Abdominal aortic aneurysms may be discovered incidentally during imaging studies or a routine physical examination as a pulsatile abdominal mass.

3. The triad of abdominal pain, hypotension, and a pulsatile abdominal mass is diagnostic of a ruptured abdominal aortic aneurysm, (the most common complication) and emergent operation is warranted without delay for imaging studies.

4. Patients with a variant of abdominal aortic aneurysm may present with fever and a painful aneurysm with or without an obstructive uropathy. These patients may have an inflammatory aneurysm that can be treated with surgical repair.

5. Other presentations of abdominal aortic aneurysm include lower extremity ischemia, duodenal obstruction, ureteral obstruction, erosion into adjacent vertebral bodies, aortoenteric fistula (i.e. GI bleed), or aortocaval

fistula [caused by spontaneous rupture of aneurysm into the adjacent inferior vena cava (IVC)].

6. Patients with aortocaval fistula present with abdominal pain, venous hypertension (i.e. leg edema), hematuria, and high output cardiac failure.

7. Patients with thoracic aneurysms are often asymptomatic. Most patients are hypertensive but remain relatively asymptomatic until the aneurysm expands. Their most common presenting symptom is pain. Pain may be acute, implying impending rupture or dissection, or chronic, from compression or distension. The location of pain may indicate the area of aortic involvement, but this is not always the case. Ascending aortic aneurysms tend to cause anterior chest pain, while arch aneurysms more likely cause pain radiating to the neck. Descending thoracic aneurysms more likely cause back pain localized between the scapulae. When located at the level of the diaphragmatic hiatus, the pain occurs in the midback and epigastric region.

8. Large ascending aortic aneurysms may cause superior vena cava obstruction manifesting as distended neck veins.

9. Ascending aortic aneurysms also may develop aortic insufficiency, with widened pulse pressure or a diastolic murmur, and heart failure.

10. Compression symptoms: Arch aneurysms may cause hoarseness, which results from stretching of the recurrent laryngeal nerves. Descending thoracic aneurysms and thoracoabdominal aneurysms may compress the trachea or bronchus and cause dyspnea, strider, wheezing, or cough. Compression of the esophagus results in dysphagia. Erosion into surrounding structures may result in hemoptysis, hematemesis, or gastrointestinal bleeding. Erosion into the spine may cause back pain or instability. Spinal cord compression or thrombosis of spinal arteries may result in neurologic symptoms of paraparesis or paraplegia. Descending thoracic aneurysms may thrombose or embolize clot and atheromatous debris distally to visceral, renal, or lower extremities.

11. Patients who present with ecchymoses and petechiae may be particularly challenging because these signs probably indicate disseminated intravascular coagulation (DIC). The risk of significant perioperative bleeding is extremely high, and large amounts of blood and blood products must be available for resuscitative transfusion.

12. The most common complications of thoracic aortic aneurysms are acute rupture or dissection. Some patients present with tender or painful nonruptured aneurysms. these patients are thought to be at increased risk for rupture and should undergo surgical repair on an emergent basis.

Investigations
Imaging Studies

1. Chest radiograph (Fig. 13.2):
   In the case of ascending aortic aneurysms, chest X-rays may reveal a widened mediastinum, a shadow to the right of the cardiac silhouette, and convexity of the right superior mediastinum. Lateral films demonstrate loss of the retrosternal air space. However, the aneurysms may also

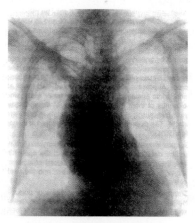

Fig. 13.2: Chest radiograph

be completely obscured by the heart, and the chest X-ray appears normal.

- Plain chest radiographs may show a shadow anteriorly and slightly to the left for arch aneurysms and posteriorly and to the left for descending thoracic aneurysms. Aortic calcification may outline the borders of the aneurysm in the anterior, posterior, and lateral views in both the chest and abdomen.

2. Echocardiography:
   - Transthoracic echocardiography demonstrates the aortic valve and proximal aortic root. It may help detect aortic insufficiency and aneurysms of the sinus of Valsalva, but it is less sensitive and specific than transesophageal echocardiography.

     Transesophageal echocardiography images show the aortic valve, ascending aorta, and descending thoracic aorta, but they are limited in the area of the distal ascending aorta, transverse aortic arch, and upper abdominal aorta. Transesophageal echocardiography can help accurately differentiate aneurysm and dissection, but the images must be obtained and interpreted by skilled personnel.

3. Ultrasonography:
   Infrarenal abdominal aortic aneurysms may be visualized using ultrasonography, but these images do not help define the extent for thoracoabdominal aneurysms.

   Carotid ultrasound may be needed for patients with carotid bruits, peripheral vascular disease, a history of transient ischemic attacks, or cerebrovascular accidents to evaluate for carotid disease.

4. Aortography:
   Aortography images can delineate the aortic lumen, and they can help define the extent of the aneurysm, any branch vessel involvement, and the stenosis of branch vessels. It describes the takeoff of the coronary ostia.

   For patients older than 40 years or those with a history suggestive of coronary artery disease, aortography helps evaluate coronary anatomy, ventricular function by ventriculography, and aortic insufficiency. It does not help in defining the size of the aneurysm because the outer diameter is not measured, which may miss dissections.

Disadvantages include the use of nephrotoxic contrast and radiation. The risk of aortography includes embolization from laminated thrombus and carries a 1 percent stroke risk.

5. Computed tomography (CT) scan:

   CT scans with contrast have become the most widely used diagnostic tool. They rapidly and precisely evaluate the thoracic and abdominal aorta to determine the location and extent of the aneurysm and the relationship of the aneurysm to major branch vessels and surrounding structures. They can help accurately determine the size of the aneurysm and assesses dissection, mural thrombus, intramural hematoma, free rupture, and contained rupture with hematoma.

   CT angiography may create multiplanar reconstructions and cines. This requires nephrotoxic contrast and radiation, but the procedure is noninvasive.

6. Magnetic resonance imaging (MRI):

   MRI and magnetic resonance angiography have the advantage of avoiding nephrotoxic contrast and ionizing radiation compared with CT scans.

   MRI and magnetic resonance angiography can also help accurately demonstrate the location, extent, and size of the aneurysm and its relationship to branch vessels and surrounding organs. These studies also precisely reveal aortic composition. However, they are more time consuming, less readily available, and more expensive than CT scans.

Other Tests

- Electrocardiogram: Baseline ECG should be performed. Transthoracic echocardiograms noninvasively screen for valvular abnormalities and cardiac function.
- Pulmonary function tests: Patients with a smoking history and COPD should be evaluated using pulmonary function tests with spirometry and room-air arterial blood gas determinations.

Diagnostic Procedures
- Cardiac catheterization: Patients with a history of coronary artery disease or those older than 40 years should undergo cardiac catheterization.

Treatment

Treatment of abdominal aortic aneurysms, thoracoabdominal aneurysms, and thoracic aneurysms involves surgical repair in good-risk patients with aneurysms that have reached a size sufficient to warrant repair. Surgical repair may involve endovascular stent grafting (in suitable candidates) or traditional open surgical repair.

Medical Therapy

All aneurysms must be treated with risk-factor reduction. Systemic hypertension probably contributes to the formation of aneurysms and certainly contributes to expansion and rupture. This is especially true of thoracic aneurysms. Strict control of hypertension is implemented in all patients, regardless of aortic aneurysm size.

Tobacco use contributes to aneurysm formation, although the exact pathophysiology is not well-understood. Cessation of smoking is recommended. Control of other risk factors for peripheral arterial obstructive disease may be beneficial.

For acute aortic dissections, All patients should be immediately admitted to an intensive care unit. Initial therapeutic goals are the elimination of pain, and reduction of systolic blood pressure to 100–120 mmHg. The first-line treatment of hypertension is with a short-acting beta-blocker (e.g. esmolol). Beta-blockade decreases the force of contraction, thus decreasing the dP/dt and shear force exerted on the dissection by minimizing the rate of rise of the aortic pressure. It also decreases the heart rate and the inotropic state of the myocardium, and reduces the likelihood of propagation of the dissection. A second-agent added is a vasodilator (e.g. nitroprusside), which reduces the systolic blood pressure too, in turn, decrease the aortic wall stress and the possibility of rupture.

Surgical Therapy
Indications

Indications for surgery of thoracic aortic aneurysms are based on size or growth rate and symptoms. Because the risk of rupture is proportional to the diameter of the aneurysm, aneurysmal size is the criterion for elective surgical repair. Elefteriades published the natural history of thoracic aortic aneurysms and recommends elective repair of ascending aneurysms at 5.5 cm and descending aneurysms at 6.5 cm for patients without any familial disorders such as Marfan's syndrome. These recommendations are based on the finding that the incidence of complications (rupture and dissection) exponentially increased when the size of the ascending aorta reached 6.0 cm (31% risk of complications) or when the size of the descending aorta reached 7.0 cm (43% risk). Patients with Marfan's syndrome or familial aneurysms should undergo earlier repair, when the ascending aorta grows to 5.0 cm or the descending aorta grows to 6.0 cm.

Rapid expansion is also a surgical indication. Growth rates average 0.07 cm/y in the ascending aorta and 0.19 cm/y in the descending aorta. A growth rate of 1 cm/y or faster is an indication for elective surgical repair.

Symptomatic patients should undergo aneurysm resection regardless of size. Acutely symptomatic patients require emergent operation. Emergent operation is indicated in the setting of acute rupture. Rupture of the ascending aorta may occur into the pericardium, resulting in acute tamponade. Rupture of the descending thoracic aorta may cause a left hemothorax.

Patients with acute aortic dissection of the ascending aorta require emergent operation. They may present with rupture, tamponade, acute aortic insufficiency, myocardial infarction, or end-organ ischemia. Acute dissection of the descending aorta does not require surgical intervention, unless complicated by rupture, malperfusion (e.g. visceral, renal, neurologic, leg ischemia), progressive dissection, persistent recurrent pain, or failure of medical management.

Patients who undergo surgery for symptomatic aortic insufficiency or stenosis with an associated enlarged aneurysmal aorta should have concomitant aortic replacement if the aorta reaches 5 cm in diameter. Concomitant aortic replacement should be consider for patients with bicuspid aortic valves with an aorta >4.5 cm in diameter.

Summary of Indications

- Aortic size
  - Ascending aortic diameter ≥5.5 cm or twice the diameter of the normal contiguous aorta
  - Descending aortic diameter ≥6.5 cm
  - Subtract 0.5 cm from the cutoff measurement in the presence of Marfan's syndrome, family history of aneurysm or connective tissue disorder, bicuspid aortic valve, aortic stenosis, dissection, patient undergoing another cardiac operation
  - Growth rate ≥1 cm/y
- Symptomatic aneurysm
- Traumatic aortic rupture
- Acute type B aortic dissection with associated rupture, leak, distal ischemia
- Pseudoaneurysm
- Large saccular aneurysm
- Mycotic aneurysm
- Aortic coarctation
- Bronchial compression by aneurysm
- Aortobronchial or aortoesophageal fistula.

Contraindications

Aneurysm surgery has no strict contraindications. The relative contraindications are individualized, based on the patient's ability to undergo extensive surgery (i.e. the risk-to-benefit ratio). Patients at higher risk for morbidity and mortality include elderly persons and individuals with end-stage renal disease, respiratory insufficiency, cirrhosis, or other comorbid conditions. For descending thoracic aneurysms, endovascular stent grafting is less invasive and is an ideal alternative (with appropriate anatomic considerations) to open repair for patients at high-risk for complications of open repair. Stent grafts are also a reasonable alternative (with the appropriate anatomy) to open repair in patients who are not at high risk for complications. Patients must understand that life-long follow-up is required and that long-term durability is unknown.

Complications

Early morbidity and mortality are related to bleeding, neurologic injury (e.g. stroke), cardiac failure, and pulmonary failure [e.g. acute respiratory distress syndrome (ARDS)]. Risk factors include emergent operation, older age, dissection, congestive heart failure (CHF), prolonged cardiopulmonary bypass time, arch replacement, previous cardiac surgery, need for concomitant coronary revascularization, and reoperation for bleeding. Late mortality is usually related to cardiac disease or distal aortic disease.

Outcome and Prognosis

Estes' 1950 report revealed that the 3-year survival rate for patients with untreated abdominal aortic aneurysms was only 50 percent, with two thirds of deaths resulting from aneurysmal rupture. operative mortality of 6–12 percent. Stroke rate varied from 3–22 percent. Renal failure that required dialysis occurred in 7 percent of patients.

Future and Controversies

Ascending aortic aneurysm repair has been well-established and is performed safely with low morbidity and mortality. The controversies lie in the use of valve-sparing root replacements in patients with Marfan's syndrome with regard to the durability of the repair. However, because most patients with Marfan's syndrome undergo the operation while they are young, they likely require reoperation eventually and the additional years of sparing their native aortic valve and living without anticoagulation are valuable.

Arch aneurysms still carry the most morbidity and mortality because neurologic injury is a great risk. Most controversies involve the methods of cerebral protection. More and more evidence suggests that antegrade cerebral perfusion is an optimal choice to reduce both temporary and permanent neurologic injury.

Recent advances in the treatment of descending thoracic aneurysms and thoracoabdominal aneurysms have used endovascular stent grafting, which offers a less invasive alternative to open surgical repair. The first FDA-approved device for descending thoracic aneurysm repair was approved in March 2005. The nonrandomized prospective comparison of open surgical versus endovascular stenting demonstrated a reduced incidence of operative mortality and reductions in paraplegia, blood loss, operative time, and length of ICU stay. The incidence of stroke between the two groups was similar.

Midterm results suggest that, although early operative mortality rates are lower with endovascular repair than with open surgical repair, late survival rates are equivalent. Paraplegia rates in the real world (as opposed to in carefully selected patient populations of clinical trials) suggest an increased incidence of paraplegia with endovascular stent grafting but range from 0–12 percent (average 2.7%).

Future studies will examine comparisons of open versus endovascular repair of thoracoabdominal aneurysms and aortic arch aneurysms.

Aneurysms are the most commonly diagnosed conditions of the thoracic aorta that require surgery. Recently, many advances in aortic substitutes, cerebral protection, and perioperative care have led to improved survival rates and outcomes.

Normal ECG

The Standard 12-Lead ECG

The standard 12-lead electrocardiogram is a representation of the heart's electrical activity recorded from electrodes on the body surface. This section describes the basic components of the ECG and the lead system used to record the ECG tracings.

1. **ECG Waves and Intervals (Fig. 14.1)**
- P wave: The *sequential* activation (depolarization) of the right and left atria
- QRS complex: Right and left ventricular depolarization (normally the ventricles are activated *simultaneously*)
- ST-T wave: Ventricular repolarization
- U wave: Origin for this wave is not clear—but probably represents "afterdepolarizations" in the ventricles

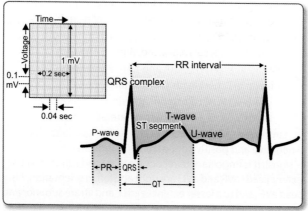

Fig. 14.1: ECG waves and intervals

- PR interval: Time interval from onset of atrial depolarization (P wave) to onset of ventricular depolarization (QRS complex)
- QRS duration: Duration of ventricular muscle depolarization
- QT interval: Duration of ventricular depolarization and repolarization
- RR interval: Duration of ventricular cardiac cycle (an indicator of ventricular rate)
- PP interval: Duration of atrial cycle (an indicator of atrial rate).

2. Orientation of the 12-Lead ECG

It is important to remember that the 12-lead ECG provides spatial information about the heart's electrical activity in three approximately orthogonal directions:

- Right ⇔ Left
- Superior ⇔ Inferior
- Anterior ⇔ Posterior

Each of the 12-leads represents a particular orientation in space, as indicated below (RA = right arm; LA = left arm, LF = left foot):

- Bipolar limb leads (frontal plane):
    - Lead I: RA (-) to LA (+) (Right, left, or lateral)
    - Lead II: RA (-) to LF (+) (Superior inferior)
    - Lead III: LA (-) to LF (+) (Superior inferior)
- Augmented unipolar limb leads (frontal plane):
    - Lead aVR: RA (+) to [LA and LF] (-) (Rightward)
    - Lead aVL: LA (+) to [RA and LF] (-) (Leftward)
    - Lead aVF: LF (+) to [RA and LA] (-) (Inferior)
- Unipolar (+) chest leads (horizontal plane):
    - Leads V_1, V_2, V_3: (Posterior anterior)
    - Leads V_4, V_5, V_6: (Right, left, or lateral)

Einthoven's triangle! Each of the six frontal plane leads has a negative and positive orientation (as indicated by the '+' and '-' signs). It is important to recognize that Lead I (and to a lesser extent Leads aVR and aVL) are right and left in orientation. Also, Lead aVF (and to a lesser extent Leads II and III) are superior and inferior in orientation. Figures 14.2 and 14.3 further illustrate the frontal plane hookup.

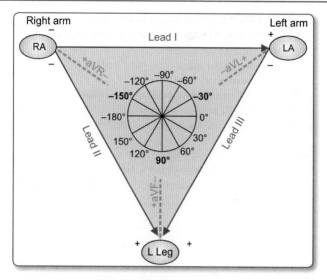

Fig. 14.2: Orientation of the 12-lead ECG

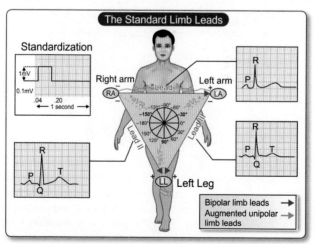

Fig. 14.3: The standard limb leads

Location of Chest Electrodes in 4th and 5th Intercostal Spaces (Fig. 14.4)

V_1: Right 4th intercostal space
V_2: Left 4th intercostal space
V_3: Halfway between V_2 and V_4
V_4: Left 5th intercostal space, midclavicular line
V_5: Horizontal to V_4, anterior axillary line
V_6: Horizontal to V_5, midaxillary line.

Analysis of ECG-A Method

This "method" is recommended when reading all 12-lead ECGs. Like the physical examination, it is desirable to follow

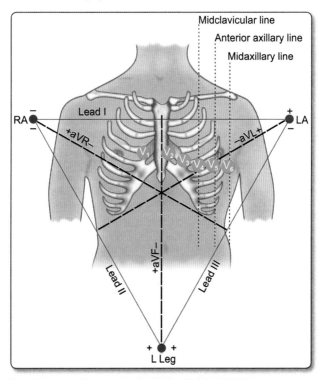

Fig. 14.4: Location of chest electrodes in 4th and 5th intercostal spaces

a standardized sequence of steps in order to avoid missing subtle abnormalities in the ECG tracing, some of which may have clinical importance. The six major sections in the "method" should be considered in the following order:

Measurements (usually made in frontal plane leads):

- Heart rate (state atrial and ventricular, if different)
- PR interval (from beginning of P to beginning of QRS)
- QRS duration (width of most representative QRS)
- QT interval (from beginning of QRS to end of T)
- QRS axis in frontal plane.

Introduction

The frontal plane QRS axis represents only the average direction of ventricular activation in the frontal plane. As such this measure can inform the ECG reader of changes in the sequence of ventricular activation (e.g. left anterior fascicular block), or it can be an indicator of myocardial damage (e.g. inferior myocardial infarction).

In the diagram below the normal range is identified (– 30° to +90°). Left axis deviation (i.e. superior and leftward) is defined from – 30 to – 90°, and right axis deviation (i.e. inferior and rightward) is defined from + 90° to + 150°.

QRS Axis Determination

- First find the isoelectric lead if there is one; i.e. the lead with equal forces in the positive and negative direction. Often this is the lead with the smallest QRS.

  The QRS axis is perpendicular to that lead's orientation.

- Since there are two perpendiculars to each isoelectric lead, chose the perpendicular that best fits the direction of the other ECG leads.

- If there is no isoelectric lead, there are usually two leads that are nearly isoelectric, and these are always 30° apart. Find the perpendiculars for each lead and chose an approximate QRS axis within the 30° range.

- Occasionally each of the six frontal plane leads is small and/ or isoelectric. The axis cannot be determined and is called indeterminate. This is a normal variant.

Examples of QRS Axis (Figs 14.5A to C)

- Axis in the normal range:
  - Lead aVF is the isoelectric lead
  - The two perpendiculars to aVF are 0° and 180°
  - Lead I is positive (i.e. oriented to the left)
  - Therefore, the axis has to be 0°.
- Axis in the left axis deviation (LAD) range:
  - Lead aVR is the smallest and isoelectric lead
  - The two perpendiculars are – 60° and + 120°
  - Leads II and III are mostly negative (i.e. moving away from the + left leg).

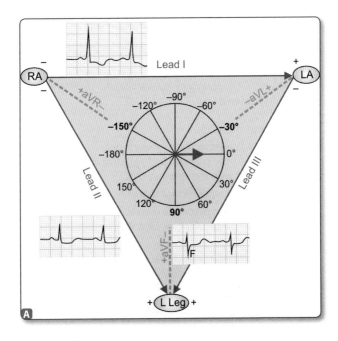

A

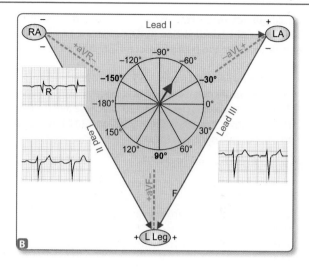

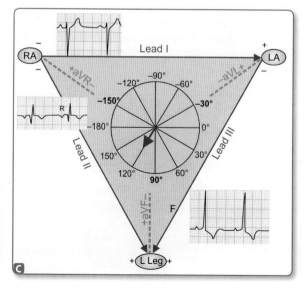

Figs 14.5A to C: QRS axis

The axis, therefore, is – 60°.

Axis in the right axis deviation (RAD) range:

Lead aVR is closest to being isoelectric (slightly more positive than negative)

- The two perpendiculars are – 60° and + 120°.
- Lead I is mostly negative; lead III is mostly positive.
- Therefore, the axis is close to + 120°. Because aVR is slightly more positive, the axis is slightly beyond +120° (i.e. closer to the positive right arm for aVR).

Rhythm Analysis

- State basic rhythm (e.g. "normal sinus rhythm", "atrial fibrillation", etc.)
- Identify additional rhythm events if present (e.g. "PVC's", "PAC's", etc.)
- Consider all rhythm events from atria, AV junction, and ventricle.

Conduction Analysis

- "Normal" conduction implies normal sinoatrial (SA), atrio-ventricular (AV), and intraventricular (IV) conduction (Fig. 14.6). The diagram illustrates the normal cardiac conduction system.

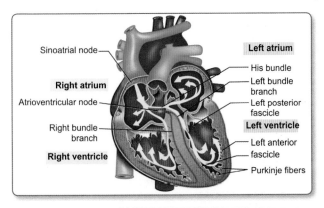

Fig. 14.6: Cardiac conduction system

The following conduction abnormalities are to be identified if present:

- SA block   : 2nd degree (type I vs. type II)
- AV block   : 1st, 2nd (type I vs. type II), and 3rd degree
- IV blocks   : Bundle branch, fascicular, and nonspecific blocks
- Exit blocks   : Blocks just distal to ectopic pacemaker site

Waveform Description

- Carefully analyze the 12-lead ECG for abnormalities in each of the waveforms in the order in which they appear: P-waves, QRS complexes, ST segments, T-waves, and... Don't forget the U waves.
- P-waves: Are they too wide, too tall, look funny (i.e. are they ectopic), etc.?
- QRS complexes: Look for pathologic Q-waves (lesson IX), abnormal voltage, etc.
- ST segments: Look for abnormal ST elevation and/or depression.
- T-waves: Look for abnormally inverted T-waves.
- U-waves: Look for prominent or inverted U-waves.

ECG Interpretation

- This is the conclusion of the above analyses. Interpret the ECG as "Normal", or Abnormal". Occasionally, the term "borderline" is used if unsure about the significance of certain findings (Fig. 14.7). List all abnormalities. Examples of "abnormal" statements are:
  - Inferior MI, probably acute
  - Old anteroseptal MI
  - Left anterior fascicular block (LAFB)
  - Left ventricular hypertrophy (LVH)
  - Nonspecific ST-T-wave abnormalities
  - Any rhythm abnormalities.

  Left anterior fascicular block (LAFB) – KH

  HR = 72 bpm; PR = 0.16s; QRS = 0.09s; QT = 0.36s; QRS axis = – 70° (left axis deviation).

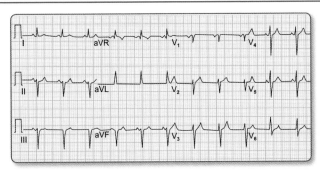

Fig. 14.7: Interpretation of ECG

Normal sinus rhythm; normal SA and AV conduction; rS in leads II, III, aVF.

Interpretation: Abnormal ECG: (1) Left anterior fascicular block.

Index

Page numbers followed by *f* refer to figure and *t* refer to table